Vegetaria
Explained

Dr. Natasha Campbell-McBride MD,
MMedSci (neurology), MMedSci (nutrition)

Vegetarianism Explained

ISBN 13: 978-0-9548520-6-1

First printed 2017

Cover photography and design by Nicholas Campbell-McBride
Illustrations by Peter Kent
Typeset by Cambrian Typesetters, Frimley, Surrey
Printed by Maple Press, York, Pennsylvania

Reviews

Dr Campbell-McBride has done it again. Her first book "Gut and Psychology Syndrome" created a small revolution in the field of Integrative Medicine. She brought forgotten cultural knowledge to the world of nutrition and the application of the content has helped tens or hundreds of thousands of autistic children to recover or improve, where all other interventions had failed.

In this well-referenced work she dares to bring even more of her common sense to the nutritional field. While we, physicians, are bombarded with one diet fad after another, pretty much every one of my patients is confused – should they be on the high protein or ketogenic diet, juicing only, high fat, no fat, vegan, raw food only, follow the China study, etc.etc. Whose advice should they follow?

As a young man I became aware that a truthful, intelligent discussion about diet in public is not welcomed. I was touched that Dr Campbell-McBride's book starts with a case related to the same issue. She brings her intelligence and uncorrupted common sense to the table and re-introduces us to the middle path of nutrition. Her recommendations are based on the observed and published truth, are easy to follow and surely will lead to greater levels of health for everyone willing to replace their belief with what actually works. It's not just a 'must-read' but also a 'must follow'!

Dr Dietrich Klinghardt, MD PhD

Since 1970 the percentage of all wildlife has reduced by an average of 57%. They're gone! Hummingbirds, elephants, rainbow trout, polar bears, honey bees,... gone. There is a mass extinction occurring that is destroying the natural world upon which humanity depends.[1]

And the same dynamic is occurring with humans. For the first time in the history of the human species our offspring are in danger of having shorter life spans than their parents. They will get sick at earlier ages, get diagnosed with diseases at earlier ages, and die at earlier ages than the age their parents die at.[2] We have to wake up! We're doing something terribly wrong!

There is a danger in our midst today. We see it in every aspect of our lives. Fanaticism (displaying very strict standards and little tolerance for contrary ideas or opinions) is permeating our governments, our spiritual and religious beliefs, and how we take care of our bodies. There is fanaticism about food, which so many people have today, that is not based on solid science.

Vegetarianism Explained is a rational, science-based, common-sense explanation of how our bodies use food, that will allow all of us – healthy people, sick people, parents raising children - to understand the role of our food choices, what different foods do in our bodies and what our bodies need. This book should be required reading for every teenager, every parent, and every person fighting an illness!

Thank you, Dr Campbell-McBride, you've produced another critical masterpiece of health guidance for us all!

Dr Tom O'Bryan, DC CCN DACBN

---

1 http://www.livingplanetindex.org/home/index
2 Olshansky SJ, Passaro DJ, et al. A potential decline in life expectancy in the United States in the 21st century. *N Engl J Med.* 2005 Mar 17;352(11):1138--45

Dr Natasha Campbell-McBride has done it again! As in her previous publications, she shone clear light where there is much misunderstanding and misinformation about nutrition and health. In this concise and cogent book she has not only explored and debunked the myths behind the putative health benefits of purely plant based diets, such as veganism and vegetarianism, but also addressed the misconception that any food, that is not animal food, is healthy. Her masterly blending of clinical cases, extensive review of the literature, and voice of personal experience make for compelling reading.

Dr Shideh Pouria, MB BS BSc MRCP (UK) PhD

Finally, a world class human digestion expert with a success resume as long as my arm explains why eating animals is positive for human health! The current diatribe against animal agriculture and meat consumption needs to tangle with a formidable foe: the human gut. As Dr Natasha Campbell-McBride dissects human digestion and its relationship to animals, the accusations that grass-fed livestock is destroying the planet are clearly disproven. Anyone who thinks the anti-livestock crowd is simply fighting for planetary peace and longevity will understand, after reading this book, that the fight is actually against the human gut. I'd like to take care of mine, thank you very much, and this book explains how to do it.

Joel Salatin, Organic Farmer, Consultant and Author, Polyface Farm, Virginia, USA

Contents

Introduction

Few things are harder to put up with than the annoyance of a good example.

Mark Twain

Vegetarianism is not common in the majority of the world's countries. Of the countries where statistics on vegetarianism (including veganism) are available, about half show less than 5% of the population. A few countries show 9–13% of the population: Austria, Australia, Israel, United Kingdom and Sweden. The remaining countries have lower numbers, apart from India, where almost 30% of the population are recorded as vegetarian.[1] India is an exception and we will talk about it in more detail in this book. However, the number of vegetarians outside India is growing, due to active promotion of vegetarianism, particularly in Western countries.

Some people decide to become vegetarian after discovering how animals and birds are treated by industrial farming. Others decide to make such a profound change in their lifestyle for emotional, political or religious reasons. Many people decide to become vegetarian because they believe that they will lose weight. Reading the promotional materials, one gets an impression that vegetarianism is the right way to live your life, that it is good for your health, kind to animals and that it saves the planet. A lot of these materials are written with an air of righteousness and aim to make the reader ashamed of eating meat. On top of that, food and nutritional sciences produce an endless number of statements proposing that meat and other animal foods are the cause of all illnesses in the world.

It is very easy to get confused! And indeed, many people do get confused. Many parents today believe that if their child decides to become a vegetarian, they must be supportive. People regard vegetarians as setting a 'good example', while vegetarians view meat-eaters with the air of a pious person looking at a sinner. Are vegetarians a good example? What about vegans? Should we all become vegetarian or even vegan? Apart from pro-vegetarian propaganda there is very little scientific information available on the subject. Amongst the small number of studies that have been done, quite a few have not been conducted very well and attract professional criticism.[2]

Thankfully, science does not have a monopoly on knowledge! Many doctors who work with vegetarian and vegan patients have accumulated valuable clinical experience. They don't need studies to tell them what effects this lifestyle can have on a person. In this book I would like to share my clinical experience and my conclusions with you, dear reader!

I hope that this book will be given as a present to anyone who is considering becoming a vegetarian or a vegan. If you care about this person, please ask them to read it first!

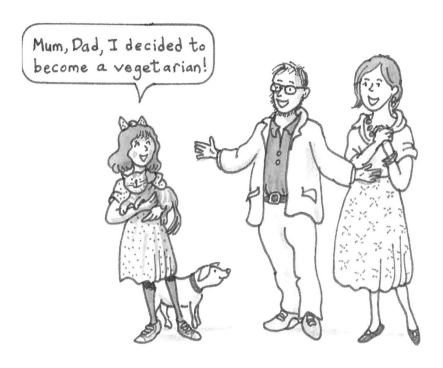

The Heart of the Matter

*Nature has taken good care that theory should have
little effect on practice.*

Samuel Johnson

Twenty-one-year-old Helen was brought to my clinic by
her worried aunt. Helen was dangerously underweight
and getting thinner by the day. She was a tall girl – 185cm
in height (over 6 feet) – with a weight of 51kg (8 stone).
She obviously used to be quite beautiful, but now she
looked emaciated and pale, her eyes were dull and her
voice feeble. Her menstruations had stopped seven
months ago.

Helen grew up abroad and came to England to study at
university. Back home processed foods were not available.
So Helen was brought up on home-cooked wholesome
meals made from fresh, locally produced ingredients;
fresh meat, fresh eggs and fresh whole milk constituted a
large percentage of her diet. She was always very healthy.
When she came to England she soon developed a dislike
for the processed junk diets her fellow students lived on,
and decided to eat a healthy diet. Brief research in popular literature led her to the idea that the 'healthiest' diet
is a vegetarian, low-fat one. So Helen started cooking her
own meals out of whole grains, beans, lentils, nuts, lots
of vegetables and fruit. She drank only water and fruit
juices. The only fat she had was some olive oil and
peanut butter. She consumed no animal foods at all and
tried to eat everything organic.

After a few months on this diet Helen's menstruations stopped and she started losing weight. But none of it seemed to worry her, as she felt 'well'. When she went home for a visit, her family were horrified by the way she looked and contacted her aunt in England to ask for help. By the time of the consultation Helen had been on her 'healthy' diet for more than a year.

So, what happened to Helen? Didn't she follow the healthiest diet in the world and the one we should all strive for? That is what some authorities and the mainstream media are telling us.

Let us try and understand the whole issue

Helen is an intelligent girl and the first good thing she did was stop eating all processed foods. These man-made concoctions wrapped in colourful packaging have no right to be called by the noble name 'food'. They are at the root of all modern epidemics of degenerative disease.[1,2,3] We will not devote any time to processed foods here; I would just sum them up with a great quote from Zoe Harcombe: 'Man is the only species clever enough to make his own food and the only one stupid enough to eat it.'[4] To have good health we need to eat foods created by Mother Nature, not man. Mother Nature took billions of years to design our bodies, while at the same time designing all the foods suitable for our bodies to use. How arrogant it is for humans to think that they know better than Mother Nature after having tinkered in their laboratories for a few decades!

Mother Nature has provided us with two groups of food: plant foods and animal foods. These two groups work differently in the body and both are important. Human beings are omnivores: we have evolved on this planet eating everything we could find in our immediate environment from both plants and animals. That is what several researchers have confirmed in their extensive study of traditional cultures around the world. The most prominent and thorough research has been conducted by Weston A. Price, an American dentist. He spent many years at the beginning of the 20th century travelling around the world to places where indigenous traditional cultures still existed. The aim of his research was to see what effect diet has on human health. At the time chronic diseases were rampant in the 'civilised' world, and it was clear that food had something to do with that. Vegetarianism was gaining popularity in America and Europe. So, when Weston A Price set off for his travels, he was specifically looking for healthy exclusively vegetarian cultures. No matter how hard he searched, he did not find one. In every corner of our planet healthy indigenous people ate a mixture of plants and animal foods, and it is the animal foods that were the most valued.[5]

Let us have a look at these two groups of natural foods in more detail.

How does it work?

All energy on our beautiful planet gets recycled, while new energy comes from the sun.[6] In order to capture the energy of the sun and convert it into solid matter Mother Nature has designed plants. Plants have a process, called photosynthesis, which captures the sunlight and converts it into chlorophyll, building the

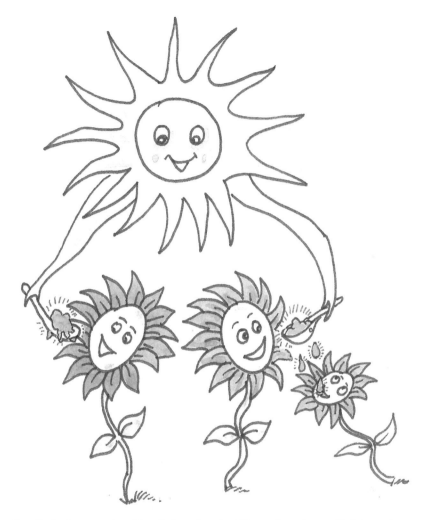

Sunlight is a major 'food' for plants. They absorb sunlight and use it for building their green mass.

plant matter. A plant in your garden can almost double in size on a sunny day! That is how efficient it is in changing the energy of the sun into solid matter, which we can touch and eat.[6]

The next group of creatures on the planet, that consume the energy of the sun in the form of plants, are herbivorous animals (animals designed to eat plant matter): cows, sheep, goats, giraffes, buffalo, elk, deer and camels.[7] Plants are generally difficult to digest.[8] The only creatures that can do it well are microbes.[9] They have incredible abilities to ferment carbohydrates, break down proteins, starch and fibre, release vitamins, and generally turn the plant matter into a form that other creatures can benefit from. This is exactly what Mother Nature used to help the herbivorous animals to digest plants and extract nutrients from them. Mother Nature equipped them with a very special digestive system, called a rumen.[7,9] It is very large, with several stomachs full of plant-breaking microbes that digest the plants for the animal.

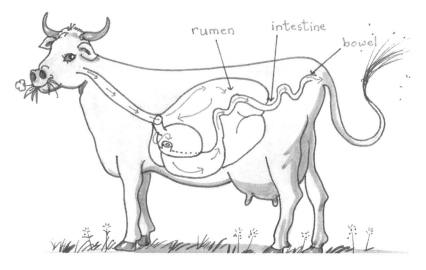

Digestive system of an herbivorous animal. The grass is digested well in the rumen first before moving into intestines, where nutrients are absorbed.

A rumen is a very busy place, where the microbes work on the plant matter (grass for example) for a while and then send it back into the mouth of the animal to be chewed again (the animal regurgitates it). After chewing the grass a bit more, the animal swallows it for further digestion. This is called chewing the cud, and an herbivorous animal can chew the same mouthful of plant matter many times, sending it back and forth between the mouth and the rumen (about 200 times in a cow!).[7] In the rumen, carbohydrates from plants get broken down, and a large percentage of them is converted into saturated fat (short-chain fatty acids – acetate, propionate and butyrate).[7,9] So the herbivorous animals are actually living on a high-fat diet, and most

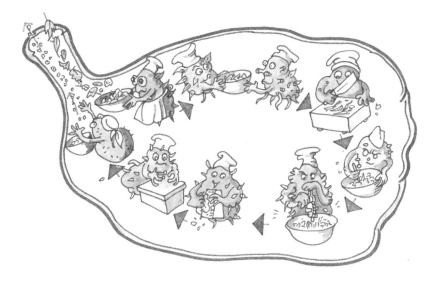

Inside the rumen. Microbes are perfectly designed to digest plants. It is not the cow that digests the grass she eats, it is microbes in her rumen that do this work for her.

of this fat is saturated. This fat is the main source of energy production for these animals.[7] The rumen has a very diverse population of microbes, including bacteria, viruses, fungi, protozoa and worms. All of these creatures participate in digesting the plant matter for the animal and converting it into a mixture of nutrients, which the animal's digestive system can absorb.[7,9] The rumen of herbivorous animals is a beautiful example of how everything in Nature works in co-operation, in harmony with each other!

In order to consume the energy of the sun in the form of herbivorous animals Mother Nature has designed the next group of life – predators. Wolves, lions, tigers, foxes, cats, dogs, etc. cannot digest plant matter, because they are equipped with a very different digestive system.[10] They can only digest meat and other animal foods. The human digestive system in its structure is similar to the gut of predatory animals: we have one small stomach with virtually no microbes in it.[11] As in predatory animals, our human stomach is designed to produce acid and pepsin, which are only able to break down meat, fish, milk and eggs. Our stomach is designed perfectly to digest animal foods! Plants, however, do not digest in our stomach to any degree; they have to wait to move out of the stomach into the intestines, where pancreatic enzymes and bile are added to the mix to break down the food further.[11] But even there the plants don't digest well. We can only break down a small part of cooked starch and absorb some juices, sugars and vitamins. The bulk of the plant – the fibre and most starch – is indigestible for the human gut.[8] It goes through the intestines and then lands in the bowel, which is the equivalent of the rumen in the human body. This is where the majority of our gut flora resides: bacteria, fungi, protozoa, viruses, worms and other creatures work on the plant matter and extract from it what they can.[12] They break down some starch

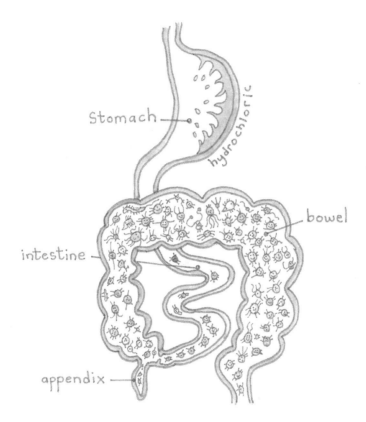

In order to digest plants we need microbes. The human stomach produces hydrochloric acid which makes it very hostile to plant-digesting microbes. In the intestines the microbial population gets gradually larger as we move closer to the bowel, where the majority of our gut flora lives. This is where plants can be digested to some degree to feed the human body.

and fibre and convert them into short-chained fatty acids, B vitamins, vitamin K_2 and other useful substances for us, the same way they do it in the rumen of herbivorous animals.

The difference between the herbivorous animals and us is that their rumen is at the beginning of their gut, while our 'rumen' – the bowel – is at the end. In herbivorous animals the plant matter is digested well in the rumen before it moves down into the part of the gut where absorption of nutrients happens. In humans the bulk of our food absorption happens higher up in the intestines, where plants cannot be digested.[8,11] So, the nutrients that we absorb in the intestines come largely from animal foods, which were digested well in the stomach. In short, the bulk of the nutrition that our bodies thrive on comes from animal foods! People knew this fact through experience for millennia. They knew that the most nourishing foods for them came from animals; they would eat plants as a supplement to meat or when animal foods were in short supply.[5]

We have been talking about natural plants: fresh vegetables and fruit, unprocessed grains, natural beans and pulses, seeds, nuts and herbs. Processed plant matter, particularly things made out of flour and sugar, has a very different digestion pattern. They have been 'pre-digested' for us by our food industry. Our gut has very little work to do to digest them, so they absorb very well and quite quickly.[11] These 'foods' are a major cause of all human degenerative diseases in the 'civilised' world.

But what about all the research published in popular nutrition books, which shows that plants are full of nourishment?[13] Yes, when we analyse different plant foods in a laboratory, they show good amounts of vitamins, proteins, fats and minerals. This information is then published in common nutritional literature, causing confusion. Why? Because, in a laboratory, we can use all sorts of methods and chemicals for extracting nutrients from plants: methods that our human digestive system does not possess.[11] The human gut has a very limited ability to digest plants and to extract useful nutrients from them. In the past, people knew that plant foods are hard for humans to digest, that is why all traditional cultures have developed methods of food preparation to extract more nutrition from plants and to make them more digestible, such as fermentation, malting, sprouting and cooking.[5] Unfortunately, in our modern world, many of these methods have been forgotten and replaced with recipes that suit the food industry's commercial agenda.

If we cook and prepare plant foods properly, can't we live on them?

That is exactly what Helen tried to do: she prepared all her food at home from natural plant ingredients. She cooked rice, oats, quinoa and buckwheat, she made her own bread, she cooked beans and lentils, she snacked on nuts and fruit and consumed lots of vegetables. Why did she get into trouble? Let us see.

The human body (without water) is largely made out of protein and fat (about half and half).[8] These are the 'bricks and mortar' from which your bones, muscles, brain, heart, lungs, liver and all other organs are made.

Laboratory analysis of plants and animal foods shows that the best protein and fat for human structure and physiology come from animal foods.[8,14,15] The amino acid profile of animal protein is correct for the human body, while the amino acid profile of plant-derived proteins is incomplete and unsuitable for human physiology. The same with fat: animal fat has the right fatty acid composition for the human body to thrive on, while plant oils are unsuitable.[15] So, when it comes to FEEDING your body and BUILDING your bodily tissues and structures, animal foods are the best and the only suitable ones!

The human body has a wonderful process, which goes on from the moment of conception until death, called *Cell Regeneration.*[11] Cells in your body (in all of your organs and tissues) constantly grow old, die and are replaced by newly born cells. This way the body maintains itself, rejuvenates itself and heals any damage. In order for your body to give birth to those baby cells, to replace the old ones, building materials are needed – proteins and fats. The best building materials to feed your cell regeneration process come from animal foods: meats, fish, eggs and dairy.[14] Growing children need large amounts of building materials for their bodies, not only for cell regeneration but for growth, so animal foods must be a very important part of their diet.[16] Apart from nutrition, animal products provide the body with energy. In fact, contrary to popular beliefs, the best source of energy for most cells in your body is fat![8,14,16]

One of the hungriest organs in the human body is the brain: it 'sponges up' around 25–45% of all nutrition floating in your blood.[8,16] Your body spends a lot of effort on feeding the brain 24 hours a day, every day.

Contrary to popular beliefs, there is much more your brain needs than just energy in the form of glucose. It is a physical organ and its cell regeneration processes require feeding with good quality protein and fat.[8,16] The brain is a very fatty organ, so it requires a lot of good quality fat to maintain its structure. On top of that, your brain manufactures neurotransmitters, hormones and hundreds of other active molecules, which are largely proteins; the brain needs building materials to make them from. The best building materials to feed your brain come from animal foods.[11,16] In the clinical practice we see degeneration of the brain function in people on purely plant-based diets: first the sense of humour goes, the person becomes 'black-and-white' in their thinking and behaviour, the sharpness of the mind goes, memory and learning ability suffer, depression sets in and other mental problems follow. These are all the signs of a starving brain.

The study of traditional indigenous people confirms the fact that animal foods are essential for us.[5] In his article about the South Seas islanders and Florida Indians, published in 1935, Weston A. Price has given a very interesting explanation of cannibalism in humans.[17] The people on the islands were divided into two groups: the coastal people, who lived by the sea and ate a lot of seafood, and the hill people, who lived high in the hills in the middle of the islands and had only plants available for them to eat. The two groups exchanged food. However, when the people from the hills did not get enough seafood for a while, their health suffered. To remedy their health problems they would come down to the coast and kill and eat coastal people. They knew from experience that the coastal people's organs (the liver in particular) had all the necessary nutrients for them, because the coastal people ate lots of fish and shellfish. They especially targeted fishermen, because people with this profession ate more seafood and their organs were particularly nutritious. Weston A. Price interviewed one fisherman who had to flee his home because he was told that the hill people had chosen him as their next victim. This example from human history shows us again that human beings cannot live without animal foods! The coastal people lived happily on their seafood; they had no thoughts about eating other people. But the hill people could not live on their plants alone; they had to supplement their diet with seafood to survive. And, when they did not get enough, they were prepared to take drastic actions.[17] This is just another example of what people are capable of when they are truly hungry. And the true hunger is always for animal foods!

Can we live on animal foods alone?

Many people would be surprised to hear that human beings can live exclusively on animal foods. In my clinic I have patients who live entirely on animal foods with great results, both children and adults. Patients with ulcerative colitis, Crohn's disease and severe mental illness do very well on a *No-Plant GAPS Diet*: not a leaf, not a speck of anything from the plant kingdom is consumed. These people live on meats, including organ meats, animal fats, meat stock and bone broth, fish (including shell fish and molluscs), fish stock, fresh eggs and fermented raw dairy – kefir, sour cream, ghee, butter, cheese and yoghurt. In some severe cases of ulcerative colitis and Crohn's disease this is the only diet that allows patients to be well, stop all medication, reach their normal body weight, eliminate all digestive symptoms and function to their full capacity. In severe cases of bipolar disorder, schizophrenia and other psychiatric conditions this diet can be a saviour! Some of these people have lived on this diet for three years or longer and have no desire to change their eating habits, because this diet works for them. Some have tried to add a little vegetable or fruit to their regimen and found that their symptoms started returning, so they had to stop.

So, based on my clinical experience, I have no doubt that human beings can live very healthily without plant foods at all!

Living entirely on animal foods is not new to our planet. Weston A. Price found that one of the healthiest groups of traditional (so-called primitive) people were Masai warriors in Africa who ate no plant matter at all.[5] They were nomadic people, travelling with their cattle, and everything they ate was provided by their animals. They ate meat, organ meats, milk and sour milk and they drank the blood of their bulls. When they were asked, why they didn't eat the fruit found in their habitat, they laughed and answered that fruit was food for their cows. These people had none of the diseases of our modern 'civilised' world whatsoever: no heart disease, no cancer, no degenerative conditions, their bodies were trim and muscular, their lifespan was long and they had beautiful healthy teeth. In addition to perfect physical health, these people were intelligent, joyful, peaceful, friendly and happy, with no psychological problems at all. But when some of them moved to a city and adopted a modern diet, they started getting the same diseases people suffer from in any modern country.[5]

So, the fact is: humans *can* live without plants! However, we cannot live without animal foods!

What are the plants for?

What about all the plant-based diets shown to help with chronic disease? Why are cold-pressed good quality plant oils shown to be beneficial for so many degenerative conditions?[18] Supplementing these oils is promoted by both the mainstream and alternative medical community. What about all the antioxidants, enzymes, vitamins, minerals, bioflavonoids and other substances in plants that are shown to be beneficial to health? Not a month passes without science discovering that broccoli has anticancer properties,[19,20] cabbage has substances that heal the digestive system,[21] nuts reduce the risk of heart disease,[22] etc., etc. Here we come to the real purpose of eating plants: they are CLEANSERS. While they are unable to feed our bodies to any serious degree, they are wonderful at keeping us clean on the inside! They also provide energy for the body to use in the form of glucose and some cofactors in the form of vitamins and minerals, but their main purpose is to keep your body clean and free of toxins. Indeed, plants in their natural fresh state are equipped with powerful detoxifying substances, which can remove various man-made chemicals, pollution and other toxins that we accumulate in our bodies.[23] Plants are particularly powerful cleansers when consumed raw. Their juices absorb in the upper parts of the digestive system, contributing a plethora of detoxifying substances and cofactors. Juicing of raw organic greens, vegetables and fruit is a major part of any cleansing protocol.[23]

When the plant matter moves further down in the gut, the fibre and starch feed the gut flora in the bowel.[24] However, the problem with fibre and starch is that they feed equally the 'bad' and the 'good' microbes. So, how good this plant matter is for the person depends on the composition of his or her gut flora. If the flora is healthy, then the fibre and starch will do you good. If your flora is unhealthy, the plant matter will feed the pathogens in your gut, which will flourish and produce many toxins and do a lot of damage. *GAPS Nutritional Protocol* is designed to normalise the gut flora and repair the gut. We remove all starch and fibre from the diet of the person in the initial stages, which is essential to allow their gut to heal.[40]

When we cook plants we reduce their cleansing ability, but make them more digestible, so they provide some building materials for the body to use. Unfortunately, these materials cannot build the body to any degree: they are largely carbohydrates, which the body uses for producing energy and then stores any surplus as fat.[16] When plants are severely processed (grains in particular) they provide the wrong materials for the body, causing disease. They overload the body with sugars, breaking some of the most fundamental mechanisms in our metabolism.[4,8] That is why consumption of products made out of flour and sugar (very processed plants) is the major cause of pretty much all degenerative health problems in our modern world: weight gain, diabetes, obesity, heart disease, cancer, Alzheimer's disease and other forms of dementia, psychological and neurological problems in children and adults, infertility, polycystic ovaries, immune abnormalities, etc.[4,16] Mounting research shows that another constituent of grains – plant proteins – is becoming positively dangerous for a growing proportion of humanity: gluten in wheat and other cereals, zein in corn, secalin in rye, hordien in barley and avenin in oats.[25,26] The reason for this is that a growing number of people have damaged gut flora. In a person with abnormal gut flora grain proteins don't digest properly and absorb in the form of peptides, which trigger chronic systemic inflammation, autoimmunity and food allergies and intolerances. Treatment of every chronic illness (from rheumatoid arthritis to cancer, and from heart disease to mental illness) must begin by removing all grains from the diet, and everything made from them.

A cleaner body always feels better than a toxic one. That is why so many people feel well on a plant-based diet in the first few weeks. One can read glowing testimonies in vegan and vegetarian books to that effect. But, when the body has finished cleansing, you need to start feeding it with animal foods. If that point is missed, the body starts starving and deteriorating. What happened to Helen? With her vegan diet she was cleansing herself, and cleansing herself, and cleansing herself, until she literally got 'washed out'. She missed the point when her body had finished cleansing and needed to start feeding. That is why she lost so much weight, despite eating large amounts of grains, beans, nuts, fruit, vegetables and vegetable oils. This 'diet', considered to be very 'healthy' in our modern society, was not feeding her to any degree!

Helen's menstruations stopped after a few months on this diet. Why did that happen? Clearly, her body was starving and conserving whatever precious resources it had left; it could not afford to waste them on monthly menstruations. But the biggest reason was lack of hormone production in Helen's body. Sex hormones are manufactured by our bodies from molecules of cholesterol.[27] There is no cholesterol in plants; it comes only from animal foods. The human body can produce cholesterol, but in a person with nutritional deficiencies the body is not able to do it efficiently. As a result, production of all steroid hormones, including sex hormones, can become low.[27,28] Without sex hormones there can be no menstruation or any other functioning of the reproductive system in humans.

This fact has been discovered and exploited by various religious orders through the centuries, because monks and nuns were not allowed to have any sexual activity. Their sexual energy was a problem for them, so they looked for ways to reduce it. They found that a plant-based diet achieved this aim very effectively: sexual desire and fertility were dramatically reduced.[29] This may be good news for nuns and monks, but for a young person, such as Helen, who is hoping to have a family one day, it is very bad news indeed! Infertility in the Western world is a big problem; many young couples are unable to produce children.[30] There is no doubt that the mainstream push for plant-based and low-fat diets is an important reason for this epidemic. Clinical experience shows that when these couples change their diet and start consuming plenty of animal foods with normal or high fat content, a large percentage of them conceive a child.[28] Recent research agrees with this observation. Researchers found that women who drink whole milk and eat high-fat dairy products are more fertile than those who stick to low-fat products. Dr Jorge Chavarro, of the Harvard School of Public Health, who led the study published in *Human Reproduction* in 2007, emphasised: 'Women wanting to conceive should examine their diet. They should consider changing low-fat dairy foods for high-fat dairy foods, for instance by swapping skimmed milk for whole milk and eating cream, not low-fat yoghurt'.[31] These high-fat foods provide good amounts of cholesterol to be converted into sex hormones, so necessary for having children.[32]

Vegan 'diets' (plant only diets) should be seen as a form of fasting. They do not feed the body properly, but provide it with a lot of cleansing. While your digestive system is busy processing plant matter (so you don't feel hungry), the diet will provide your body with large amounts of cleansing substances. The ultimately toxic people are cancer victims; they require a lot of cleansing. That is why many nutritional cancer treatment protocols are vegan.[23] However, if followed as a permanent lifestyle, veganism often leads to developing cancers, because the body simply runs out of resources to look after itself.[33] When your body has finished cleansing it will need feeding, and that is when you have to introduce animal foods. If that is not done the body starves, starts cannibalising itself and problems start developing. What happened to Helen is a good example of that.

When visiting India I met some Hindu pilgrims travelling to their sacred religious sites. Part of their pilgrimage is a 41-day fast, which they described as 'very difficult'. They are not allowed to eat any animal foods at all and live entirely on plants – vegetables, fruit, rice, lentils and beans, nuts, vegetable oils and bread – precisely the Western vegan 'diet'. These people consider it to be a *fast*, not a diet, and do it very rarely as part of a religious pilgrimage. So, when talking about purely plant-based eating the word 'diet' should not be used, instead such a regimen should be called a *Vegan Fast*. One cannot fast forever. Like any other form of fasting, veganism can only be used as a temporary measure to cleanse the body. It must never be chosen as a permanent lifestyle!

Vegetarian diets that include animal foods can be adopted as a long-term strategy. It is possible to be a healthy vegetarian, as long as you continue eating some animal foods to provide feeding/building substances for your body, such as plenty of eggs and full-fat dairy. Obviously all processed foods should be removed and the diet needs to be natural. Such vegetarian cultures exist in India. People there understand just how valuable animal foods are for them. That is why the cow is considered to be a sacred animal in India – she provides milk, butter, cheese and ghee. Apart from cows, people in India keep goats and highly value their milk. Many vegetarians in India also keep chickens and ducks and consume plenty of fresh eggs. Many consume meat and fish when they can get them.

There are many forms of vegetarianism: some eat fish, some eat eggs and dairy, some allow occasional consumption of meat. People who get into trouble are those who decide to stop eating meat and live largely on processed foods. They get ill very quickly. This group of people is particularly prone to diabetes, obesity, heart disease and cancer.[34]

Another group of people who get into trouble are those who follow low-fat vegetarianism. A lot of impetus for removing fats from the diet comes from counting calories, because fats produce the highest amount of calories per gram.[35] The idea that you can equate Mother Nature's food to calories is a shameful indictment on nutritional science! Food is not a calorie; it is a million times more complicated and interesting. The human body is not a furnace for burning calories either – it is also a million times more complex. Looking at food in terms of calories is just another example of how lost and inadequate our food science is. Human beings cannot live without fats![27,28,32,35] Mother Nature took billions of years to design our foods and everything she put into them is essential, including fat. Every component in a natural food is balanced with all other components; they work as a whole. To remove fat from a natural food is to make it incomplete and unbalanced; the human body cannot thrive on such 'food'. Low-fat vegetarianism typically leads to degenerative diseases of the nervous system and immunity. Mental illness, particularly anorexia nervosa, is one of the very common results of this regimen.[28,32,36]

Let us summarise this chapter

There are two groups of natural foods on our beautiful planet, and each of them has its own role to play in human physiology.

Animal foods (meat, fish, eggs and dairy) are largely building/ feeding foods. They feed the cell regeneration in the body, allowing the body to maintain its normal physical structure and chemical composition. In other words, animal foods provide the 'bricks and mortar' your body is made from. Apart from that, your body manufactures a myriad of protein-based chemicals every day – hormones, enzymes, neurotransmitters and others – that are essential for your body to function. In fact, your body can be seen as a chemical factory of sorts. The raw materials this factory needs come from animal foods. Animal foods are particularly important for growing children, as their bodies need large amounts of building materials for growth and development. These foods are absolutely essential for a pregnant woman to consume, because she is building a body for her baby. Building materials are needed for that, and the mother must do her best to provide the best building materials she can find. Following a vegan fast during pregnancy can be absolutely disastrous for the child and the mother. But even vegetarianism where parents eat dairy products and eggs may not provide optimal nutrition for the child. I have seen a number of vegetarian families in my clinic, where children suffered from autism, diabetes type one, allergies, anaemia and many other health problems. In all cases, the children were malnourished and the parents were malnourished too.

Plant foods (grains, beans, fruit, vegetables, herbs, nuts and seeds) are good foods for cleansing and detoxifying, but they do not feed the body to any serious degree. They keep the body clean on the inside by helping it to remove toxins and wastes. They provide energy for the body in the form of glucose. They provide some microelements for the body to use: minerals, vitamins, phytonutrients and cofactors. They feed the gut flora in the bowel and allow it to produce many useful nutrients for us: B vitamins, vitamin K_2, short-chain fatty acids and other useful substances. However, plant foods cannot be used successfully as the only source of food.

Of course, this division is not black-and-white, there is some overlap: animal products, particularly raw, have a considerable cleansing ability while plants have some feeding ability, particularly when cooked, fermented and sprouted.[37,38,39]

So let us enjoy both the animal foods and the plant foods, working in harmony for our bodies! The important thing is to keep them natural with minimal processing. In order for us to find the best quality natural foods, we must know where our food comes from. In the next chapter we are going to look at how food is produced in our modern world, and the implications of plant-based diets for our Planet Earth.

Where Does Your Food Come From?

We don't inherit the Earth from our ancestors,
we borrow it from our children.

David Brower

For the majority of people in the Western world their food comes from a supermarket. Our supermarkets are groaning with inexpensive food, giving us a feeling of abundance. Where does all this food come from? How is it produced? At whose expense is it produced? How can they afford to sell it so cheaply? Is it good quality? Many people are starting to ask these questions. They also wonder why, with such an abundance of food, we have growing statistics of degenerative diseases in the population?[1]

Food is big business! A myriad of commercial and political interests are involved at every step of food production and distribution. As a result, our world is full of commercial misinformation about food. On top of that, we have food science, largely funded by commercial companies, which is producing an endless stream of nutritional misinformation for the population.[2] Because it is 'science', people believe it. To find true information about food takes a special effort.

There is a myth perpetuated in the media that we cannot produce enough meat, milk and eggs to feed the population.[3] This idea comes from industrial farming, where animals and birds are raised in factories (CAFOs – Confined Animal Factory Operations) in terrible conditions.[4] They are crowded to the point that the animals cannot turn around, they stand and sleep in their own waste and are fed commercial feed, inappropriate for their physiology. The waste from these confinement operations is a toxic pollution poisoning our waterways.[3,4,33] And the meat, eggs and milk produced are of poor quality. Animals and birds kept in confinement are prone to diseases and require constant input of expensive antibiotics and other drugs.[4] On top of that, government regulations are difficult to comply with.[9] So animal husbandry is not popular amongst industrial farmers. Growing plants, however, is much easier for a conventional farmer because of modern machinery and chemicals; and Western governments subsidise growing of crops.[5] So indeed, from the point of view of industrial agriculture, growing crops is much easier than producing meat, milk and eggs.

However, when it comes to truly organic, natural food production, the truth is just the opposite – producing meat, milk and eggs is easy compared to producing plant foods. All you have to do is provide natural, ecologically clean habitat for the animals and birds to live in. As a result they are healthy and do not need much extra feeding or care.[6] All cows, sheep, goats and other herbivorous animals need is natural chemical-free pasture with plenty of growing grasses and herbs. They will convert this plant matter into meat and milk for us. And the grass grows for free! All you have to do is keep moving the animals to new pastures to allow grasses to recover after grazing.[7] The same goes for birds: they need organic pasture to roam on, and they will find a lot of their own food – worms, grubs, grasses and herbs.[8] As they roam, the animals and birds fertilise the land, helping it to build new layers of humus-rich topsoil and increasing diversity of grasses and herbs in the pasture, improving its quality year after year.[6,8]

What is difficult to produce naturally is plant matter: vegetables, grains and other edible plants. The reason for this is that growing plants naturally involves a lot of hard work, and the yield is unpredictable, because the produce is prone to damage by weather, birds, disease, animals and insects.[9] Nature does not grow monocultures – fields of one plant species. In any natural meadow there are dozens of species of grasses and herbs growing in a mixture, supporting each other and protecting each other from diseases and pests.[9] We, humans, want to grow wheat on one field, lettuce on another and so on. As this idea goes against Nature, these monocultures are prone to diseases and pests. So chemicals are heavily applied to get these monocultures to survive. Ask any organic or biodynamic farmer, or even a person who grows their own organic vegetables in a garden, and they will tell you that growing plants naturally is difficult and very labour intensive.

Organic plants do not keep well; that is why organic produce has to be local and seasonal. With a few exceptions, truly organic vegetables and fruit will not travel around the globe well and then look 'fresh' on a supermarket shelf. Organic produce also doesn't 'look good' to an average consumer: the fruit and vegetables are all different sizes and can have blemishes and spots on them. Supermarkets do not accept this kind of produce, because their customers want their vegetables and fruit to look 'perfect'. As the demand for organic produce increased, industrial agriculture wanted a piece of the pie.[10] As a result, they have watered down organic standards.[11,12] A lot of produce labelled 'organic' in supermarkets today is likely to come from these companies. On top of that, unfortunately, there is also a lot of cheating in the organic sector, when non-organic produce is sold as organic.[11] To eat truly organic fruit and vegetables we have to grow them ourselves or get them from local organic producers, who usually sell their produce themselves or through small distributors.

In the last couple of decades vegetarianism has been vigorously promoted in the mainstream media, with claims that it will 'feed the growing population', that it is 'kind to animals', 'will save the planet' and that it is 'a healthy lifestyle'.[13] The fact is, the only way to support populations of vegetarians is through chemical industrial agriculture![14] Only by using machines and toxic chemicals we can produce the yield of plant matter necessary. This propaganda for vegetarianism has likely been launched by the agrochemical industry, which can increase their profits dramatically if large populations of people turn vegetarian. Plant matter produced by industrial agriculture is full of pesticides, herbicides and other highly toxic chemicals.[15] There is no health to be gained by eating large amounts of these plants!

Arable industrial agriculture uses cultivation methods and chemicals that destroy the soil.[16,17] The soils of arable fields in the Western world are so damaged today that most of them are unable to support any plant life at all without the application of chemicals.[17] Many old farmers will tell you that in their childhood and youth there were worms in the soil on their fields and crops grew without any chemicals. Now there are no worms or any other signs of life in the soil and nothing would grow on it without chemicals.[16]

The topsoil on our planet is a source of all life! It is the most precious part of Nature and it is being lost in staggering amounts every year due to the activity of our arable industrial agriculture, busy growing plants for us to eat.[16,17,18] There is nothing 'saving the planet' in choosing a vegetarian lifestyle, just the opposite: you become an activist for the destruction of the planet!

Many people don't know that healthy topsoil is one of the most concentrated sources of carbon on Earth.[17]

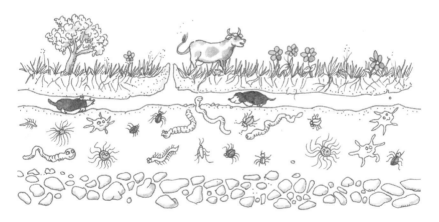

Healthy soil is a community of many life forms, from tiny viruses, bacteria, fungi, protozoa and other microbes, to worms, insects, mice and moles. These creatures create humus-rich fertile top soil in co-operation with grazing animals and plants. It is a balanced eco-system and all life on Earth is based on it.

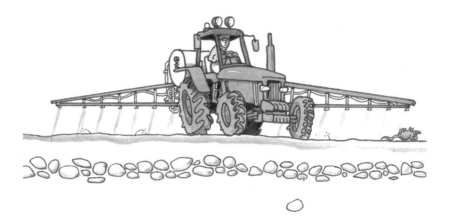

Industrial agriculture destroys top soil. The soil becomes thin and loses its living community, turning into dust which is not able to support any life or hold water.

As the soil gets destroyed, the carbon is released into the atmosphere. Industrial arable agriculture is a major contributor to global warming on our planet – probably the biggest contributor![17,18] Environmental scientists have already calculated that if we converted even a fraction of arable fields in the West into organic pasture, we would remove large amounts of carbon from the atmosphere by locking it in the soil, and reducing or even eliminating the threat of global warming as a result.[19] Animals are essential in maintaining the health of topsoil on our planet. As they graze on pasture they build layers of carbon-rich topsoil.[17,18,19] By increasing the numbers of pastured animals on the planet we can remove excessive carbon from the atmosphere! But, of course, the companies which profit from industrial arable agriculture work very hard to suppress this information and prevent this from happening. Instead, they have put out false propaganda that animals 'belch out methane' and increase global warming.[17] This nonsense doesn't withstand common sense, let alone any scientific assessment.[20]

Amongst all the human activity on Planet Earth industrial agriculture causes the biggest damage to our environment.[16,17,18,19] It is an established fact that all deserts on the planet have been created by human activity, including the Sahara, Gobi, Nevada and Australian deserts.[16,18] Arable agriculture destroys the soil, turning it into dust. The Great Plains of America are a good example of that.[17,18,21] When Europeans first reached that vast area of the American continent they saw herds of buffalo so large, that they stretched to the horizon.[20] In the following decades people killed the buffalo and turned the Great Plains into arable fields. The buffalo, over centuries, had built thick layers of topsoil, so the yields of crops were high for some years. But as the soil was destroyed, the yields reduced to nothing. The dead soil turned to dust and was blown away towards the Pacific Ocean. Once fertile, the Great Plains of America were turned into a dust bowl, a semidesert.[17,18,20]

Healthy soil holds large amounts of water.[22,23] Destroyed or damaged soil has no ability to hold water. The rains run off these fields and cause flooding in nearby villages and towns.[17,18,23] In Europe and other industrialised countries, every winter thousands of people suffer from flooding, which is becoming more intense every year. We have to thank arable industrial agriculture for that. Having destroyed the soil, agricultural chemicals leach into ground waters and poison our water supply.[24] Chemical analysis of standard water supplies in Western countries shows the constant presence of these chemicals. Our water companies know that these chemicals are unavoidable and have developed 'acceptable levels' of these poisons in our drinking water.[25] Numbers of research studies have found that animals, insects and other life forms, which live in rivers and streams around arable fields, are becoming extinct or damaged by the agricultural chemicals. In addition, numerous small animals are killed by agricultural machines every year, while others disappear because their habitat has been destoyed.[17,26] So there is nothing 'kind to animals' or 'kind to the planet' in a vegetarian lifestyle, because it has to rely on arable industrial agriculture.

Our planet is paying a very heavy price for all the plants we are growing on an industrial scale. Who benefits from that? Somebody very powerful – commercial companies which produce agricultural chemicals and machinery. At one of my presentations to an American organisation of organic farmers I mentioned that one of the biggest agrochemical companies in their country influences their government. As soon as I said that, several people from the audience shouted: 'They *are* our government!'. Indeed, these very wealthy companies infiltrate governments of Western countries and guide their policies on food and agriculture.[27] The greed of these companies is never ending: no matter how much profit they produce this year, they must produce more the next year. How can they do that? By selling more chemicals and machinery to the farmers. How can they do that? By creating more arable lands and more demand for plant matter. In order to do that they have created propaganda for vegetarianism, and a slogan 'We must feed the planet!', which our government officials are parroting to the population. Yet, every year, our industrial agriculture *overproduces* grain![17,28,29] This fact is carefully hidden, while the media gives people the idea that we are not producing enough. So governments dictate that more land should be ploughed, more pasture and forest should be converted to arable fields and more grain should be grown.[17,30] All this is done in order to increase the profits of the agrochemical commercial complex.

What about the animals and birds? As their pasture is converted into arable fields to grow more grain, they are confined to prisons – factories, where they are fed that overproduced grain.[31] Grain is not an appropriate food for cows and other herbivorous animals; it makes them ill.[30,32] Mother Nature has designed them to eat grass on pasture. Industrial agriculture is focussed on profit, not on the health and well being of animals and birds. So, the animals and birds spend a short miserable life in confinement, eating inappropriate food for their physiology; then they are slaughtered and sold as meat in supermarkets.[31,33] As the demand for grass-fed meat has grown, our industrial agriculture has found a way to deceive the consumer, and Western governments happily approved it. Animals are locked up in confinement and fed grass, which is harvested from fields sprayed with chemicals.[30] The grass is usually one or two species of hybrid grasses, which do not grow on natural pasture because they cannot survive without chemical fertilisers.[30,32] They call these animals 'grass-fed' and sell their meat at a premium in supermarkets as 'grass-fed meat'.

This kind of meat cannot be compared to meat from animals and birds that spend a happy healthy life on real natural pasture, eating foods that Mother Nature has designed them to eat.[30,32] People who have started raising their own animals and birds naturally will tell you that never again will they want to eat meat, milk or eggs from a supermarket. Having tasted meat, eggs and milk of proper quality – the quality Mother Nature has intended for us – they do not want to tolerate the poor quality of industrially produced food again! Eggs are a good example. Commercial egg producers use feed for their chickens that contains synthetic dye to make the egg yolks yellow.[34] Without this synthetic dye the yolks will be too pale to be acceptable. Eggs from chickens that range free on organic pasture obtain their colour from carotenoids and other natural substances in the grasses and herbs that chickens eat in abundance.[32] Apart from grass, free-range chickens eat lots of meat in the form of worms, grubs and insects – very good sources of protein and natural fats for the chicken. An egg is almost pure protein and fat, so chickens need a good amount of these nutrients in their diet. Commercial feed for chickens and other animals claims to provide protein in the form of soy. But soy is indigestible for most animals, including humans.[35] Only microbes can digest it – a fact well known in traditional Japanese and Chinese culture, where soy has always been fermented to make food from it. Fermentation is applying microbes to break down food, to pre-digest it for us. Chickens fed exclusively on commercial feed produce inferior quality eggs compared to chickens on pasture.

Many people who choose to become vegans make this choice after discovering how industrial farming treats animals and birds. The cruelty of the system puts them off eating animal foods. But is becoming a vegan the right way to fight that system? What you do is exactly what industrial agriculture wants you to do – eat more plants! By no longer eating animal foods you play directly into their hands, while damaging your own health.[46] The right thing to do is not to stop eating meat, eggs and dairy, but to start buying them from organic natural farmers! These farmers treat their animals with love and care; they provide them with natural habitat to live in and feed them food natural to their physiology.[32] These are happy and healthy animals and birds. The food we get from them is healthy and nourishing. These are the farmers and the animal welfare system that we all must support! Unfortunately, governments in the Western world do not support natural organic farmers, instead they support industrial agriculture. It is very difficult to survive running a natural farm nowadays; those farms that do well, do so thanks to the consumers who support them.

What about milk? Milk used to be considered Nature's perfect food. For millennia, to have a cow in the family was a blessing and a basis for the good health of the whole family.[36] Unfortunately, our industrial agriculture was not happy with the amounts of milk a normal cow can produce. They wanted more milk to increase their profit. So Western scientists have come up with a

solution – they created a new breed of cow in a laboratory. Today we have a large black-and-white cow, which
can produce three times more milk per day than a
normal cow is able to produce.[37] These animals are not
natural, they cannot survive on grass only and have to
be fed grain, soya and many other additives.[30] These
cows are unhealthy: about 75% of them have mastitis at
any time, so antibiotics are routinely given to them in
food (these antibiotics finish up in milk).[30] They suffer
from arthritis, infertility and cancer, and the majority of
them die at an early age.[37] An unhealthy animal
produces unhealthy milk! Almost all milk and dairy
products in Western supermarkets today come from
these cows. No wonder medical science has accumulated a large amount of data to show that this milk is a
causative factor in every degenerative disease on the
planet: from heart disease, mental illness and autoimmune problems to cancer.[38]

Fortunately, there is a consumer movement in the
Western world for *real* milk, from natural breeds of cow
fed on organic pasture.[39] Many farmers are producing
this excellent quality milk today and it is sold raw,
unpasteurised. Western governments, ruled by the
commercial world, have created different laws and regulations for the sale of this kind of milk. In some places
it is banned, in other places can be sold at farmer's
markets only or at the farm gate.[40,41] But the good news
is: if consumers want to have real natural milk, they can
get it in most places in the Western world today! The
commercial milk industry has tried very hard to
pronounce raw (unpasteurised) milk 'dangerous', claiming that it can carry infections. Research shows that raw

milk is very safe to drink. In fact it is better protected from infections than pasteurised milk.[42,43,44] Milk is almost the white blood of the animal with some cells removed. It is full of alive, active immune cells, white blood cells, enzymes, hormones, probiotic microbes and other elements, which protect it from infections.[45] When we pasteurise milk, we kill it. It becomes a dead substance which cannot protect itself from any microbe. Of course, any food can get contaminated, including milk. However, modern organic farming follows very strict hygiene practices, so there is no risk of having infections that people used to get from milk some hundred years ago (tuberculosis, for example).[44] Infected milk comes from an infected cow. All animals in the Western world are regularly tested for infections and the veterinary standards are very high. So, having raw milk from an organic pasture-fed cow today is very safe; safer than it has ever been.

In conclusion

So, dear reader! What do you choose: industrial chemical agriculture or organic natural food production? Poor quality food, full of agricultural chemicals and antibiotics, or real food? If you choose vegetarianism, please reconsider! Your choice spells disaster for our planet, because it is based on industrial arable agriculture. Only this kind of agriculture will be able to produce all the plants you want to eat. If you are a person that works hard in the garden to produce your own plant matter, then that deserves respect. However, people who grow their own organic vegetables will tell you that it is not possible to produce enough organic plant matter in a private garden to feed even one vegetarian for a year! That is why vegetarians buy their food in supermarkets, even those who have organic gardens. Industrial agriculture is rapidly becoming the most powerful destructive force for our planet. It destroys the topsoil, releasing carbon into the atmosphere and causing global warming. It poisons land and water and produces disease-causing 'food' for us – food, based on suffering animals and birds and chemically produced plants, which are forced to grow on exhausted deficient soils. Food that destroys our beautiful planet. And food that ultimately destroys us!

Why not choose the natural way of producing food? Instead of the arable wasteland that our countryside has become today, imagine land with many pastures and herds of healthy and happy animals. After a few years of rotational grazing the animals will restore the land's fertility, so we can grow some healthy organic crops on this land. Imagine pigs raised in a forest (a perfect environment for them), where they can eat acorns and roots, grubs and caterpillars, grasses and leaves – their natural food – and assist the forest in its growth and good health. Imagine flocks of chickens raised in organic orchards, where chickens dig and eat grubs and caterpillars, protecting the trees, while fertilising the ground. These orchards will produce excellent organic fruit without any chemicals. Imagine geese and ducks raised in swampy areas and on pasture near ponds and lakes, where they will help the soil to build rich humus, which holds large amounts of water. This will protect nearby villages and towns from flooding and give the birds a happy healthy habitat to live in. Our food can be produced in harmony with Nature without damaging the Planet, but instead making it even more beautiful and plentiful!

Unfortunately, this kind of change can never come from above, because we are ruled by the commercial and political machine. This kind of change can only come from the grass roots – individuals who make a conscious choice about what they want to eat, and how they want their food to be produced. The more farms diversify and convert to organic and natural, the better our food supply will become. Only organic diversified farms, where animals and birds are given a chance to restore the fertility of the land so we can grow healthy crops on it without any chemicals, can provide the real quality of food we all want. Find these farms and support them! Buy their produce exclusively! When you buy directly from the farmer, your food will be less expensive, fresh and excellent quality. The result will be better health and vitality for you and your loved ones.

There is no good health without good food!

There is no good food without healthy soil!

And there is no healthy soil without happy and healthy farm animals and birds!

Food, Glorious Food!

Let food be thy medicine and medicine be thy food!

Hippocrates, 46–370 BC

Misguided vegetarianism and veganism are becoming an important cause of physical and mental illnesses in our modern world.[1,2] Due to mainstream propaganda, the majority of the population believes that it is healthy to be a vegetarian. Many young people become victims of this propaganda. It is possible to be a healthy vegetarian, but one has to know what one is doing. It is easy to develop multiple nutritional deficiencies and get into trouble, if you don't know how to feed your body properly. Typically these youngsters don't do any research and start living on pasta, sugar, bread, cakes and other processed carbohydrates. The typical result of this kind of vegetarianism is gaining weight, because processed carbohydrates cause the body to store food as fat. So, the next step for many young vegetarians is low-fat vegetarianism or even veganism. It doesn't take long for their immune system to collapse, and the person starts getting one infection after another, followed by many courses of antibiotics. Antibiotics destroy the person's gut flora with many serious consequences. The person develops *GAPS – Gut And Psychology Syndrome* and *Gut And Physiology Syndrome*. Anorexia nervosa, depression, bipolar disorder, obsessive-compulsive disorder and other mental illnesses usually follow. Physically the person can develop digestive disorders, allergies and food intolerances, migraines, arthritis, chronic cystitis, hormonal problems and autoimmune disease. To understand the whole picture, let us have a look at the case history of a girl called Hanna (the name has been changed). I have described this story in my book *Gut And Psychology Syndrome*.[3] Her story is very typical.

Hanna was a healthy child until the age of 13: she did well at school, played sports, had friends and was almost never ill. She had never had antibiotics in her life and was breastfed as a baby for a year. At the age of 13 she decided to become a vegetarian, which her parents did not object to. From that point on her diet consisted of breakfast cereals, pasta, rice and a lot of bread and potatoes. However, she was OK because she ate eggs and full cream dairy and was not concerned about how much fat was in her food. Around 16 years of age she went to a dancing school, where she was put under pressure to lose weight. In order to lose weight, she decided to become a vegan and stopped eating anything with any fat in it. In a matter of a few weeks she got glandular fever, which was treated with a long course of antibiotics. The glandular fever lasted a year, and Hanna still feels that she has not recovered from this infection fully. From 17 she went through almost constant throat and chest infections, treated with antibiotics. At 18 she went to university, where she decided to become a model, so she had to lose weight again. In order to do that she started taking laxatives and slimming pills. This went on for two years, she became painfully thin, grew very weak physically, was constantly ill with infections and colds, her menstruations stopped, her digestive system was in a poor shape (she developed constipation alternating with diarrhoea, nausea, vomiting, bloating, abdominal pain and indigestion) and she became depressed. The diagnosis of anorexia nervosa followed and Hanna had psychotherapy and counselling. Her problems led to a conflict with her parents, who were desperate to help her, but all their efforts were sabotaged by Hanna. She continued with her very poor diet (low fat vegetarianism), laxatives and all sorts of slimming pills. By 19 she felt suicidal and took an overdose of paracetamol. This led to regular hospitalisations in psychiatric facilities, psychiatric medications and repeated suicidal attempts.

As you can see, Hanna was a healthy child before she decided to become a vegetarian. Her parents believed that vegetarianism was a healthy lifestyle and allowed their 13-year-old daughter to make such a life-changing decision without any study or preparation. As a result, their daughter has destroyed her health and her life! Unfortunately, her story is becoming more and more common.

What kind of information should Hanna have been given before being allowed to become a vegetarian? What kind of things should her parents have known? Let us go through this information. A lot of what we will talk about in this chapter I have already described in detail in my previous publications. However, this information is so important that it makes sense to repeat it here.

THERE IS NOTHING IN THE WORLD MORE POWERFUL IN ITS EFFECT ON HUMAN HEALTH, THAN FOOD!

We eat at least three times a day, sometimes more often. Every morsel of food you eat changes your metabolism and your health. Western health systems are crumbling under the burden of chronic disease, physical and mental. The numbers of people who are chronically ill are growing all the time, and many illnesses are becoming younger (people get them at a younger age, than they used to in the previous generations). The first and most important cause of these illnesses is consumption of processed foods.

Let us talk about it in more detail.

Processed foods

We live in an era of convenience foods, which are very processed foods. When Mother Nature made our human bodies, she at the same time provided us with every food we need to stay healthy, active and full of energy. However, we have to eat these foods in the form that Nature made them. It is when we start tampering with natural foods that we start getting into trouble. Any processing that we subject the food to changes its chemical and biological structure. Our bodies were not designed to have these changed foods! The more food is processed, the more nutrient depleted and chemically altered it becomes.[1,2,4,5] Apart from losing its nutritional value, processed food loses most of its other properties: taste, flavour and colour. To compensate for that, various chemicals are added:

flavour enhancers, colours, various E numbers and other additives.[1,2,3,4,5] Many of these chemicals have been conclusively shown to contribute to inflammation, cancer, memory loss, hyperactivity and learning disabilities, psychiatric disorders and other health problems.[6,7,8,9,10,11]

Natural foods do not keep very long, so industry changes them to prolong their shelf life. To achieve that, natural foods are subjected to extreme heat, pressure, enzymes, solvents and countless numbers of various other chemicals; fats are hydrogenated, carbohydrates are modified and proteins are denatured.[1,2,3] In the process, natural foods are changed into various chemical concoctions, which are then packaged nicely and presented to us as 'food'. 'Food' that is made to suit commercial purposes where health considerations never enter the calculation. The manufacturers are obliged to list all the ingredients on the label. However, if the manufacturer uses an ingredient that has already been processed or is made from processed substances, this manufacturer is not obliged to list what that ingredient was made from.[2,3] So, if you are trying to avoid something in particular, like sugar or gluten, for example, reading an ingredient list may not always help you.

If we look at supermarket shelves, we will see that the bulk of processed foods are carbohydrates. Breakfast cereals, crisps, soft drinks and beer, biscuits, crackers, breads, pastries, pastas, chocolates, sweets, jams, condiments, sugar, preserved fruit and vegetables and frozen precooked meals with starches and batter are all highly processed carbohydrates. When we eat them, they put the body in a fat-storing mode, which causes weight gain and obesity; our obesity epidemic in the world is caused by processed carbohydrates.[12,13] They create chronic systemic inflammation in the body, leading to heart disease, diabetes, cancer and many other chronic degenerative conditions.[13]

Processed carbohydrates have a direct effect on our behaviour and are addictive. They get absorbed very quickly, producing an unnaturally rapid increase in blood glucose.[12] A rapid increase in blood glucose, called **hyperglycaemia**, puts the body into a state of shock, prompting it to pump out lots of insulin very quickly to deal with the excessive glucose.[12,13] As a result of this overproduction of insulin, about an hour later the person has a very low level of blood glucose, called **hypoglycaemia**. Have you ever noticed that after eating a sugary breakfast cereal in the morning you feel hungry again in an hour? That is hypoglycaemia. What do people usually have at that time in the morning to satisfy their hunger? A biscuit, a chocolate bar, a coffee or something like that, and the whole cycle of hyper-hypoglycaemia begins again. This up and down blood glucose roller-coaster is extremely harmful for anyone, children and adults alike. It has been proven that mood swings, lethargy, hyperactivity, inability to concentrate and learn, aggression and other behavioural abnormalities in children and adults are a direct result of this glucose roller-coaster.[14,15,16,17] The hyperglycaemic phase produces the feeling of a 'high', with hyperactive and manic tendencies, whilst the hypoglycaemic phase makes us feel unwell, often with a headache, bad mood, aggression and general fatigue.

Another important point about processed carbohydrates is their detrimental effect on the gut flora.[18,19] Processed carbohydrates feed pathogenic bacteria and fungi in the gut, promoting their growth and proliferation. In addition to that they make a wonderful glue-like environment in the gut for various worms and parasites to take hold and develop.[20,21] Many of these microbes and creatures produce toxic substances that go into the bloodstream and literally 'poison' the person.[22,23] By negatively altering the gut flora, processed carbohydrates also play an important role in damaging the person's immune system, because gut flora is a major regulator of the immune status. And, as if that is not enough, processed foods (particularly processed carbohydrates and sugar) directly weaken the functioning of macrophages, natural killer cells and other immune cells, and undermine systemic resistance to all infections.[17,21,22,23,24] People who have sugary drinks, crisps, sweets, breakfast cereals and other processed foods daily worsen their immune system's condition by these food choices.

Let us have a look at some of the most common forms of processed carbohydrates.

Breakfast cereals

They are supposed to be healthy, aren't they? That is what numerous TV advertisements tell us. Unfortunately, the truth is just the opposite.[17,25,26]

- Breakfast cereals are highly processed carbohydrates, full of sugar, salt, trans fats and other unhealthy substances. A bowl of breakfast cereal will start your day with the first round of the blood sugar roller-coaster, with its all too familiar symptoms for you to deal with.

- Being a great source of processed carbohydrates, breakfast cereals feed pathogenic bacteria and fungi in the gut, allowing them to produce their toxins.

- What about fibre? The manufacturers claim that with a bowl of their product you will get all the fibre you need. Unfortunately, it is the wrong kind of fibre for the majority of people. Fibre in breakfast cereals is full of phytates – substances that bind essential minerals and take them out of the system, thus contributing to mineral deficiencies, which can lead to osteoporosis and other problems.[27] On top of that, fibre from grains contains lectins, substances that can damage your digestive system and the rest of the body.[28,29,30]

- There has been an interesting experiment performed in one of the food laboratories. They analysed the nutritional value of some brands of breakfast cereals and the paper boxes in which these cereals were packaged. The analysis showed that the box, made of wood pulp, had more useful nutrients in it than the cereal inside.[31] Indeed, breakfast cereals have got a very low nutritional value. To compensate for that, the manufacturers fortify them with synthetic forms of vitamins, claiming that by eating your morning bowl of this cereal you will get all your daily requirements of those vitamins. Well, the human body is not that simple; it has been designed to recognise and use natural vitamins that arrive in natural food form. That is why synthetic vitamins have a very low absorption rate, which means that most of them go through and out of your digestive tract without doing you any good.[32] Whatever vitamins do get absorbed, the body often does not recognise as food, so they get taken straight to the kidneys and excreted in urine.

So, no matter what the advertisements say, there is nothing healthy in breakfast cereals for any of us.

Crisps, chips and other starchy snacks

Crisps, chips and popcorn, the backbone of children's diet nowadays, are highly processed carbohydrates with many detrimental effects on the human body. But that is not all: they are soaked with vegetable oil that has been heated to a very high temperature. Any plant oil that has been heated contains substances called trans fatty acids, which are unsaturated fatty acids with an altered chemical structure. They replace the vital omega-3 and omega-6 fatty acids in the cellular structure, making the cells dysfunctional. Consuming trans fatty acids has a directly damaging effect on the immune system. Cancer, heart disease, eczema, asthma and many neurological and psychiatric conditions have been linked to trans fats in the diet.[33]

Recently, another strong argument appeared against consuming crisps, chips and other processed carbohydrates – the acrylamides.

The acrylamides story

In the spring of 2002 the Swedish National Food Administration and Stockholm University reported that they had found highly neurotoxic and carcinogenic substances in potato crisps, French fries, bread and other baked and fried starchy foods. These substances are acrylamides.[34,35] Scientists in Norway, UK and Switzerland have confirmed this finding. They have also found acrylamides in breakfast cereals and other starchy foods that have been fried or baked at high temperatures. Recently, instant coffee has been added to the list of foods containing these highly dangerous substances. The World Health Organisation, United Nations Food and Agriculture Organisation and the US Food and Drug Administration have developed a plan to identify how acrylamides are formed in foods and what can be done to eliminate them, since they can cause cancer, neurological damage and infertility. Acrylamides are so harmful to health that there are certain maximum limits set for these substances in food packaging materials.[34,35] For years government agencies paid a lot of attention to controlling the amount of acrylamides in plastic food packaging, but nobody looked at the food inside that packaging. Now it has been discovered that some foods inside these plastic packets have incredibly high amounts of acrylamides – way above all allowed limits.[35,36] The acrylamides story provides another reason for us to avoid crisps, chips, other starchy snack foods, bread, breakfast cereals and instant coffee.

Wheat

Virtually nobody buys wheat as a grain and cooks it at home; we buy foods made out of wheat flour. Wheat flour is the main ingredient in most processed carbohydrates. The flour arrives at bakeries in pre-packaged mixes for different kinds of breads, biscuits and pastries. These mixtures are already processed, with the best nutrients lost. Then they are 'enriched' with preservatives, pesticides to keep insects away, chemical substances to prevent them from absorbing moisture, colour and flavour improvers and softeners, just to mention a few. The bakery makes breads, pastries, cakes, biscuits, etc., from these chemical cocktails for us to eat, adding more processed ingredients on the way. Wheat flour digests and absorbs very quickly and will overload your system with glucose. For example, a slice of a typical white bread will give you the equivalent of about five teaspoons of sugar, which goes quickly into your bloodstream, leading to a condition called metabolic syndrome.[37] This condition lays the ground in the body for developing obesity, heart disease, diabetes, cancer, autoimmune disease and many other maladies. Wheat flour is present in most processed foods. It has become so pervasive in Western culture that the majority of us don't realise just how much of it we consume on a daily basis. We eat wheat cereal and toast for breakfast, sandwiches and baguettes for lunch, pasta for dinner and biscuits and cakes in between: about 70 to 85% of everything entering many people's mouths daily is wheat.[31] Our physiology has not been designed to consume so much of one particular substance at the expense of everything else! People know that they should consume more fruit and vegetables, but the problem is that their stomachs are filled with wheat all day long and there is no room left for fruit and vegetables. As almost 100% of wheat products are highly processed foods, it is wheat that makes up the bulk of our health-damaging processed diets today. There is no doubt that foods made from wheat flour are a major contributor to every degenerative disease on this planet.[31,32]

Sugar and anything made with it

Sugar was once called a 'white death'.[37] It deserves 100% of this title. The world consumption of sugar has grown to enormous proportions in the last century – 171 million metric tonnes.[38] Sugar is everywhere, and it is hard to find any processed food without it. Apart from overloading the body with glucose and causing metabolic syndrome and blood glucose roller-coaster, and having a detrimental effect on the gut flora, it has been shown to have a directly damaging effect on the immune system.[24,37] Sugar is considered to be the most addictive substance on the planet. A large percent of the Western population is addicted to sugar. Sugar addiction is the basis for developing all other addictions (drugs, alcohol, tobacco, dangerous behaviour, etc).[37,44] When we eat sugar, to deal with it the body has to use available minerals, vitamins and enzymes at an alarming rate, finishing up by being depleted of these vital substances.

Let us see how that happens.

In order to metabolise only one molecule of sugar, your body requires around 56 molecules of magnesium, dozens of molecules of vitamins, enzymes, minerals and other nutrients.[24,32,37,39] When we analyse a piece of fresh sugar cane or sugar beet in their natural state in a laboratory, we find that every molecule of sugar in them is indeed equipped with 56 molecules of magnesium and all those other nutrients.[40,41] So, when we eat natural sugar cane and sugar beet without processing them, the sugar in these plants gets used by the body well and brings us only health. But we do not eat sugar beet or sugar cane in their natural form. We extract the sugar out of them and throw everything else away. That pure sugar comes into the body like a villain, like a highway robber pulling nutrients out of our bones, muscles, brain and other tissues in order to be metabolised.[24,32] It needs those 56 molecules of magnesium! Where is all that magnesium going to come from? From your bones, your muscles and other organs. Consumption of sugar is a major reason for the widespread magnesium deficiency in our modern society, leading to high blood pressure, heart attacks, strokes, neurological, immune and many other problems.[42,43] And this is only magnesium we have discussed. What about all the other nutrients that will be depleted in your body as a result of eating sugar? Their deficiencies will bring you many other symptoms and health problems.[44]

Cakes, sweets, and other confectioneries are made with sugar and wheat flour as the main ingredients, plus lots of chemicals (colours, preservatives, flavourings, etc.). It goes without saying that they should be out of the diet if we are to prevent every modern disease.

Soft drinks (pops, cordials, lemonades, etc.) are a major source of sugar in our modern diets, not to mention chemical additives. A can of soda can contain from 5 to 10 teaspoons of sugar.[45] Consumption of soft drinks is one of the main reasons for our epidemics of metabolic syndrome and obesity, particularly in children. When we are thirsty our bodies need water, not sugary, chemical concoctions in colourful bottles. Commercial fruit juices are no better: they are full of processed fruit sugars and moulds.[46] Unless freshly pressed, they should not be in our diet either. While we are talking about drinks, it makes sense to mention beer. Beer is made from grains and sugar and is full of partially broken-down starch. It presents your body with a double whammy of highly processed carbohydrate in combination with alcohol. It causes metabolic syndrome in the body: the so-called 'beer belly' is one of the signs of this disorder. Consumption of beer is a major factor in obesity, diabetes and heart disease epidemics.[37,44,45] So, if we would like to avoid those disorders, we have to make beer consumption very occasional.

As people become aware of the harmful effects of sugar on health, the industry keeps coming up with various new chemical sweeteners and puts them into food production using powerful marketing tools. It usually takes science a few years to find out about their damaging effects on health. A good example is saccharine. It had been on the market for decades before science found that it causes cancer.[47] Another example is aspartame, a sugar replacement in so-called 'diet' drinks. It has been found to be carcinogenic and neurotoxic; it has been particularly implicated in our epidemic of multiple sclerosis.[48,49,50,51] Another modern sweetener is high fructose corn syrup (HFCS). Despite the fact that it has been proven to cause just about every chronic disease on the planet, it continues to be used extensively by the food industry in processed foods and soft drinks.[52,53] It is best to avoid all man-made sweeteners as they are not natural to our physiology. Mother Nature gave us good healthy sweeteners, which we will discuss later.

Processed fats

All margarines, butter replacements, spreadable butter, vegetable oils, cooking oils, hydrogenated oils, shortenings and many other common fats are processed fats, which are alien to our human physiology and must not be consumed if we want to avoid every modern degenerative disease.[54,55] You will find processed fats in most processed foods: breads and pastries, chocolates, ice cream, biscuits, cakes, pre-prepared meals, crisps, snacks, popcorn, sauces, mayonnaise, condiments, all fried foods, baby formula, vegetarian foods, etc.

The basis of all processed fats are vegetable oils.[56] Vegetable oils are extracted from plants. All plant oils contain very fragile polyunsaturated fatty acids, which are easily damaged by heat, light and oxygen.[54] That is why Mother Nature has hidden them away very carefully in the cellular structure of plants – in their oily seeds, leaves, stems and roots. When we eat plants in their natural form we get these oils in their pristine state and they are very good for us. But when we take plants to our big factories and extract the oils from them, something very different happens. Very high temperatures, pressure and various chemicals are employed, which change the structure of fragile fatty acids in the plant matter creating a plethora of unnatural, chemically mutilated, harmful fats.[54,56] Then these chemically mutilated oils are put into bottles and sold in supermarkets as cooking oils and vegetables oils, and added to all processed foods.

From the very beginning of these oils appearing in the human food chain worried scientific studies started coming out demonstrating that industrial vegetable oils cause cancer, heart disease, diabetes, neurological damage, infertility, immune abnormalities and other health problems.[57,58,59,60,61] These oils are full of chemically changed fatty acids, which our human bodies are not meant to have!

Many of these changed fats in vegetable oils have not even been studied yet and we don't know what havoc they can wreak in the body. However, a group called trans fats has received a great deal of attention.[62,63,64] These are unsaturated fatty acids whose chemical structure has been changed through processing. Trans fatty acids are very similar in their structure to their natural counterparts, but they are somewhat 'back to front'. Because of their similarity they occupy the place of essential fats in the body, while being unable to do their jobs. That, in a way, makes cells disabled.[54] All organs and tissues in the body are affected. For example, trans fats have great immune-suppressing ability, playing a detrimental role in many different functions of the immune system.[62] They have been implicated in diabetes, atherosclerosis, cancer and neurological and psychiatric conditions.[62,66] They interfere with pregnancy and conception, the normal production of hormones, the ability of insulin to respond to glucose and the ability of enzymes and other active substances to do their jobs.[62] They have damaging effects on the liver and kidneys.[62] A breast-feeding mother would have trans fats in her milk fairly soon after ingesting a helping of a 'healthy' butter replacement.[54,62] A baby's brain has a very high percentage of unsaturated fatty acids; trans fats would replace them and interfere with the brain development. There is simply no safe limit of trans fats in the diet. And yet a packet of crisps will provide you with about 6g of trans fats, a small snack packet of cookies will give you 7–12g, a snack packet of processed cheese (mainly advertised to children) will provide 8g of trans fats, a tablespoon of a common margarine will give you 4–6g, a portion of French fries, cooked in vegetable oil will serve you with 8–9g of trans fats.[54,64] Given their ability to impair bodily functions on the most basic biochemical levels, there is no doubt that their role in our modern epidemics of degenerative disease is greatly underestimated. Trans fats and other processed fats can directly cause immune problems, infertility, heart disease, cancer, diabetes, mental illness and many other health problems.[65,66]

In order to make vegetable and cooking oils look solid and prolong their shelf life, they are hydrogenated.[63] Hydrogenation is a process of adding hydrogen molecules to the chemical structure of oils under high pressure at a very high temperature – 120–210^{0}C (248–410^{0}F) – in the presence of nickel, aluminium and sometimes other metals. Remnants of these toxic metals stay in the hydrogenated oils, adding to the general toxic load, which the body then has to work hard to get rid of.[54] Hydrogenation of vegetable oils creates products which are even more toxic and harmful to health.

Consumption of large amounts of vegetable and cooking oils presents another problem for the body: the excess of omega-6 fatty acids.[55,67] To be healthy our bodies require a very delicate balance between different fatty acids. When we eat plants in their natural state the oils we consume from them do not upset that balance. But when we eat processed foods full of vegetable cooking oils we receive excessive amounts of omega-6 fats, which contribute to a pro-inflammatory environment in the body and lead to disease.[54,55,67]

Processed salt

Only a small percentage of all industrial salt production goes for human consumption. More than 90% of all salt produced is used for industrial applications: the making of soaps, detergents, plastics, agricultural chemicals, PVC, etc., etc.[82] These industrial applications require pure sodium chloride. However, salt in Nature contains many other elements: in fact natural crystal salt and whole sea salt contain all the minerals and trace elements that the human body is made of.[84,85] In this natural state salt is not only good for us, but essential. Because the industry requires pure sodium chloride, all other elements and minerals are removed from the natural salt. We consume it under the name of 'table salt' and of course all our processed foods contain plenty of it.[84]

This kind of salt upsets our homeostasis on the most basic level.[88,91] Our bodies have been designed to receive sodium chloride in combination with all the other minerals and trace elements that a natural salt would provide.[83,84,85] Pure sodium chloride draws water to itself and causes water retention, with many consequences such as high blood pressure, tissue oedema and poor circulation.[87,89] As the body tries to deal with the excess of sodium chloride, various harmful acids and gall bladder and kidney stones are formed.[86,87] As sodium in the body works in a team with many other minerals and trace elements (potassium, calcium, magnesium, copper, zinc, manganese, etc.), the levels of those substances get out of normal balance.[84,87,90] The harmful results of table salt consumption can be numerous and very serious. That is why most medical practitioners, including mainstream doctors, tell us not to consume table salt.

Our planet has plenty of good quality salt for us to consume. Throughout human history, salt has been highly valued: it used to be called 'white gold'; the Roman Empire paid its soldiers with salt (hence the word 'salary').[83,85] Natural salt is just as fundamental to our physiology as water is.[92,93] We need to consume salt in its natural state: as a crystal salt from salt mines or as whole unprocessed sea salt. There are a number of companies around the world that can provide you with good quality natural salt.

No soya, please!

Soya is very big business, particularly in the USA. A large percentage of the industry uses genetically modified soya.[68] Soya is cheap to produce and, following some questionable research showing that it can be beneficial for menopausal women, the market has exploded with soya products. Soya can be found in many processed foods, margarines, salad dressings and sauces, breads, biscuits, pizza, baby food, children's snacks, sweets, cakes, vegetarian products, dairy replacements, infant milk formulas, etc. Is there a problem with that? Let us have a look at some facts.

1. In Japan and other eastern cultures soya is traditionally used as a whole bean or fermented as soy sauce, tofu, natto, miso and tempeh.[69] The form in which soya is used in the West is called *soy protein isolate.*[70] How is it made? After removing the fibre with an alkaline solution, the soya beans are put into large aluminium tanks with an acid wash. Acid makes the soy beans absorb aluminium, which will remain in the end product.[68] Aluminium has been linked to dementia and Alzheimer's disease, and indeed there has been a lot of publicity recently that links soya consumption with these mental disorders.[71,72] After the aluminium-acid wash the beans are treated with many other chemicals, including nitrates, which have been implicated in cancer development. The end product is an almost tasteless powder, easy to use and add to any food. The majority of processed foods contain this powder, and of

course soya milk, yoghurt and infant formulas are made out of it.[68] It is a highly processed substance with poor nutritional value and a lot of harmful qualities. Animals fed this product die from cancer and malnourishment and produce sick offspring.[68,73] Recently its consumption has been linked to cancer, autism, inflammation and other degenerative conditions in humans.[68,73,74,75]

2. Soya is a natural goitrogen. What does this mean? It means that soya has an ability to impair thyroid function. Low thyroid function has very serious implications for your health, including inability to lose weight, depression, poor immune function, heart disease and many other problems.[68,73,75,76]

3. Soya beans have a very high concentration of phytates. These substances are found in all grains as well, particularly in their bran. Phytates have a great ability to bind to minerals, which prevents them from being absorbed, particularly calcium, magnesium, iron and zinc.[68,77,78]

4. Soya has gained its popularity as a treatment for menopause because it contains plant oestrogens, which do not work in the body in the same way as their natural counterparts do. It is questionable whether these substances are indeed useful for menopausal women. For the rest of us, particularly for men and children, they are most definitely harmful. There is growing concern among health professionals about the quantity of plant oestogens infants and small children might be getting from soya milk and infant formulas.[76,79,80]

5. Western producers of soy would like you to believe

that the health of Japanese people depends on their consumption of soya. The truth is very different. Soya in Japan is consumed largely in a fermented form and in small amounts.[81]

If you want to eat soya, have it only in the natural, traditional fermented form as soy sauce, natto, miso, tofu and tempeh. These foods are prepared according to traditional wisdom, which has served people in the East for centuries. Vegetarians who consume meat replacements made out of soya must study this information and understand what they are doing to their bodies.

What should we eat to be healthy and full of energy?

Let's start with shopping. Buy your food in the shape and form that Nature has made it and prepare it yourself at home, using traditional methods of cooking: on the stove, the grill or in the oven. Avoid microwaves, as they destroy food and can make it carcinogenic.[1,2]

What should we buy?

1. Buy meats, fresh or frozen, including game and organ meats.
Avoid all mainstream processed meats: hams, bacons, sausages, delicatessen, tinned meats, etc. because they are full of preservatives and other chemicals that have been proven to cause illness.[4,5] Meats prepared in a traditional way using natural salt and fermentation are

safe to eat and taste much better (traditional hams, sausages and salami). Avoid genetically modified meats. Our physiology has been designed to have meats as Nature designed them – without antibiotics, pesticides and other chemicals. Look for natural pasture-fed meats, preferably organic. Avoid lean meats; our physiology can only use meat fibres when they come with the fat, collagen and other substances that a proper piece of meat will provide.[3] When we eat poultry it is important to eat the skin and the fats, as well as the meat; and the most valuable nutrients come from the legs, wings, skin and carcase of the bird, not so much from the breast.[6] If you want sausages, find a local butcher who will make them for you on order with just minced meat (full fat), salt, pepper, chopped onion and any fresh herbs of your choice. Order them in bulk and keep them in the freezer. Once you have tasted these sausages you will never want to eat the commercial ones again (full of wheat and chemicals). Contrary to popular belief, it is meats, fish and other animal products that have the highest content of vitamins, amino acids, nourishing fats, many minerals and other nutrients which we humans need on a daily basis.[3] All this nutrition in meats and fish also comes in the most digestible form for us humans. I find it deceptive when vitamin tables in some books on nutrition show that plant foods (grains, vegetables, fruit, etc.) provide all our vitamins. First of all, the form in which plants contain these vitamins is difficult for us to digest. Secondly, if you compare the amounts of vitamins in meat, fish or other animal products with plant foods, it is the animal products that are at the top of the list. Let us have a look at just some of them.[3,7]

Vitamin B1 (thiamin): the richest sources are pork, liver, heart and kidneys.

Vitamin B2 (riboflavin): the richest sources are eggs, meat, milk, poultry and fish.

Vitamin B3 (niacin): the richest sources are meat and poultry.

Vitamin B5 (pantothenic acid): the richest sources are meat and liver.

Vitamin B6 (pyridoxine): the richest sources are meat, poultry, fish and eggs.

Vitamin B12 (cyanocobalamin): the richest sources are meat, poultry, fish, eggs and milk.

Biotin: the richest sources are liver and egg yolks.

Vitamin A: the richest sources are liver, fish, egg yolks and butter. We are talking about the real vitamin A, which is ready for the body to use. You will see in many publications that you can get your vitamin A from fruit and vegetables in the form of carotenoids. The problem is that carotenoids have to be converted into real vitamin A in the body, and a lot of us are unable to do this conversion, because we are too toxic, or because we have an ongoing inflammation in the body.[8] So, if you do not consume animal products with the real vitamin A, then you may develop a deficiency in this vital vitamin despite eating lots of carrots. Vitamin A deficiency will lead to impaired immunity and development of any chronic illness in the body.[7,8,9]

Vitamin D: the richest food sources are fish liver oils, eggs and fish.

Vitamin K2 (menaquinone): the richest sources are organ meats, full-fat cheese, good quality butter and cream (yellow from grass-fed animals), animal fats and egg yolks. This vitamin is essential for our health, its deficiency leads to deposition of calcium in the soft tissues and initiation of inflammation.[10] Apart from the high fat foods, an important source of this vitamin is our own gut flora: the probiotic bacteria in the gut produce and release vitamin K2. Fermented foods contain vitamin K2 as the bacteria produce it in the process of fermentation; natto (fermented soy beans) is one of the richest sources in Eastern culture while in the West well-aged natural full-fat cheese is a good source of this vitamin. [9,10]

All these vitamins are absolutely essential for us, humans; we cannot live without them, let alone function well. Three well-researched vitamins, which are generally thought to come from plants, are vitamin C, folate and vitamin K1 (phylloquinone). However, now we know that liver contains good amounts of both vitamin C and folate.[7,9] Combining meats and fish with vegetables in your meals will provide you with the full spectrum of nutrients.

Organ meats (liver, kidney, heart, brain, tongue, etc) have been considered to be a delicacy and the most valuable food in all traditional cultures.[11] These foods contain concentrated amounts of nutrients. Fresh liver is an absolute powerhouse of nutrition for our physiology and should be consumed on a regular basis, particularly by people with nutritional deficiencies. People with anaemia should have fresh liver and red meats daily (lamb, beef, game and organ meats in particular) because these foods are the best remedy for anaemia.[3,8] Not only do they provide iron in the haem form, the form that the human body absorbs best, but they also provide the B vitamins and other nutrients essential for treating anaemia. Meats also promote better absorption of non-haem iron from vegetables and fruit, while vitamin C from vegetables and greens promotes absorption of iron from meats.[3,9] Large epidemiological studies show that eating red meat is associated with a much lower incidence of iron deficiency and anaemia in various countries of the world.[3]

The mainstream misinformation about meats, particularly red meats, has been driven by commercial powers, which profit from replacing these natural foods with their processed alternatives. Fresh, natural meats have nothing to do with heart disease, cancer or any other disease, and are important for us to eat in order to provide all the nutrients we humans need.[12,13]

Home-made meat stock is a wonderful nutritional and digestive remedy, something our grandmothers used to make on a daily basis. The best stock is made from bones, joints and offcuts. All you have to do is boil them on a low heat for 2–3 hours in water, with some salt and pepper added. As you cook bones, joints and meats in water, the nutrients from them get extracted into the water. The resulting stock is rich in collagen, gelatine, minerals, amino acids and many other nutrients, which have a healing effect on your digestive system, your joints, your brain, your immunity and the rest of your body.[12,14] Use these meat stocks for making soups, stews and simply as a warming therapeutic drink with and between meals. Chicken stock made from a whole chicken is the best remedy for a cold or a tummy upset. It goes without saying that all commercially available stock granules and cubes are to be avoided. They do not possess any of the healing properties of a home-made meat stock and are full of detrimental ingredients. Meats cooked in water are easier to digest for a person with a sensitive digestive system.[15]

2. Buy fish and shellfish fresh or frozen.
Avoid tinned, cooked, dyed and other processed fish and shellfish. Wild fish is always better than farmed. There is a question, however, about mercury and other pollutants that we pump into our oceans and rivers. For that reason, some official bodies recommend limiting fish consumption.[16] However, research shows that people who consume more fish are in better health than people who limit it.[17] A healthy human body has a good ability to handle pollutants and remove them. The first and the best barrier to any pollution coming with food is healthy gut flora.[18] The beneficial bacteria in our gut flora have an excellent ability to bind, neutralise and remove from the body mercury, lead and other heavy metals and toxins. However, in people with damaged gut flora these poisons remain in the body, so restoring normal gut flora is very important, particularly after a course of antibiotics.[19] To limit your exposure to environmental toxins it makes sense to avoid large carnivorous fish, such as tuna, shark and swordfish, as they accumulate more pollutants than small fish.[20,21] Smaller fish, such as oily fish (sardines, mackerel and herring) and any other wild fish, are important for us to eat on a regular basis. They provide us with

good proteins, minerals and essential fats. Fish oils are the best anti-inflammatory remedies Nature has given us and they work best when consumed as part of the whole fish.[22,23]

3. Buy fresh eggs from free-range hens, preferably organic. Eggs are a wonder food, full of easy-to-digest nutrition. A fresh, raw egg yolk is absorbed literally without needing digestion and provides you with almost every nutrient under the sun in the best possible biochemical form.[24] In the pre-antibiotic era raw eggs were traditionally used as a cure for tuberculosis because they provide powerful immune-boosting nutrients.[26] Any person with memory loss must have at least three, preferably five to six, fresh eggs a day. It has been demonstrated in a number of clinical trials that eating fresh eggs improves memory.[25] Learning ability and behaviour in children can be improved tremendously by consumption of fresh eggs.[28] Children should have at least two eggs a day. The faulty hypothesis that fats and cholesterol 'cause' heart disease has scared people away from eating eggs because they contain cholesterol. Cholesterol is one of the most important substances in the human body. The story that it 'causes' heart disease is an absolute fallacy; cholesterol is an essential-to-life substance, and eating dietary cholesterol is no more harmful than drinking water.[27] Please read a full description of cholesterol's role in human health in my book *Put your heart in your mouth. What really causes heart disease and what we can do prevent and even reverse it.* It goes without saying that you must avoid any processed eggs: dried egg powders, mixes, etc. Fresh eggs are an excellent food for breakfast, cooked any way you like. Served with a fresh salad and plenty of cold-pressed virgin olive oil, eggs will set your blood sugar and body biochemistry at a normal level for the day.

4. *Buy fresh vegetables, not frozen, tinned, cooked or other-wise processed.*

French artichoke, beets, asparagus, broccoli, Brussels sprouts, cabbage, cauliflower, carrots, cucumber, celery, marrow, courgette (zucchini), aubergine (eggplant), garlic, onions, kale, lettuce, mushrooms, parsley, green peas, peppers of all colours, pumpkin, squash, spinach, tomatoes, turnips, watercress and other low-starch vegetables are your best choices.

Those of you who grow your own organic vegetables know that they do not keep even two days; as soon as you pick them they start wilting. So, how do all the vegetables in our supermarkets look 'fresh' for weeks? The industry washes them in chemical solutions to preserve them, even organic vegetables. Every time we eat these vegetables we eat chemicals. This particularly applies to greens (spinach, salad leaves, lettuce, etc). The only solution to this problem is to have your own organic garden! Not only will it provide you with wonderful food, but you will spend more time in the fresh air and sunlight communing with Mother Nature.

There is a mountain of information available on the benefits of eating vegetables, as they contain a plethora of wonderful nutrients.[24,28] They should be eaten every day, both cooked and raw. Cooked vegetables are easier to digest and provide warm nourishment for the body, while raw vegetables keep our bodies clean inside as they provide powerful detoxifying substances and the best quality fibre.[28] In cold weather and when you have a cold, eat plenty of warming soups and stews with well-cooked vegetables. Cold salads do not agree with our physiology in those conditions. However, in hot weather cold salads are exactly what we need. The best vegetables come from people's private gardens: fresh, in season and usually organic. Vegetables that have to travel half across the world to reach your table are not in the same league in any possible way.

Try to replace wheat products, such as bread, pasta, pastries, pies, biscuits, etc., with vegetables and your body will reward you in a matter of days with better health, more energy, clearer thinking and good sleep.[24,25,28]

5. Buy fresh fruit, not cooked, tinned, frozen or processed in any way.
Fruit needs to be ripe! Unripe fruit is difficult to digest. You have to understand that anything you cannot digest properly will do you no good. Unfortunately a lot of fruit in your supermarket is likely to be unripe.

Sweet and tropical fruits should be consumed between meals as they may interfere with the digestion of meats.[25] The exceptions are avocado, tomato, lemon and other fruits that do not taste sweet. People who have abnormal gut flora often cannot digest different fruits, and have to avoid them. Once you take steps to improve your gut flora, you may be able to eat fruits that you could not tolerate before. Just like vegetables, the best fruit comes from people's private gardens – fresh, organic, picked ripe and full of nutrients. Commercially produced fruit is likely to be sprayed with chemicals, picked unripe and grown on exhausted soils. Organic is always better than non-organic. I know a lot of people who could not tolerate various fruit and vegetables until they switched to their organic counterparts.

Berries are a wonderful variety of fruit, absolutely packed with cleansing nutrients.[24,25] Raspberries, black, red and white currants, gooseberries, elderberries, blackberries, strawberries, etc. are full of vitamins, antioxidants, minerals and many other substances that will regulate your blood sugar level and keep your body clean on the inside. Regular consumption of *uncooked* fresh or frozen berries will prevent heart disease, cancer and many other maladies.[28,29] Take any chance to pick your own berries in season and freeze them for the winter. When you want to have jam, just defrost some berries and mix them with honey to taste. Make just enough to consume in a few days because this jam will not keep for long.

6. Buy natural organic dairy.
Unprocessed milk, unprocessed cream, fresh natural butter (not spreadable and not butter substitutes), natural ghee, natural live yoghurt, kefir and natural cheeses produced in a traditional way. Avoid all processed cheeses, dried and long-life milk and cream, and other long-life or processed dairy.

One processing that most commercial milk is subjected to nowadays is homogenisation, when the milk is forced through a fine mesh to break down the fat globules. This is done purely for cosmetic purposes and takes the milk one more step away from its natural state, making it more processed.[32,33] It is particularly important to stick to organic dairy, as milk accumulates most chemicals that non-organic cows are exposed to.[31]

Dairy products are full of wonderful nutrition and are important for us to eat.[24] However, a lot of people cannot tolerate milk. This is because commonly available milk has been pasteurised. Pasteurisation destroys milk: it changes the chemical structure of its proteins, fats and carbohydrates, kills beneficial bacteria and destroys enzymes and vitamins.[30,36] Pasteurised milk is difficult for most of us to digest, particularly infants and children. That is why milk allergy and intolerance is so common. Unprocessed, unpasteurised, straight-from-the-cow milk is very easy to digest as it contains enzymes that digest the milk for you to some degree.[34,35] However, this milk must be organic and should come from natural breeds of animals. Non-organic cows often have mastitis, so a lot of pus and infectious organisms finish up in their milk. This kind of milk has to be pasteurised.[31] Organic pasture-fed cows are healthy and their milk is free from infections; it does not need pasteurisation. There is a growing number of farmers around the world who produce organic, unprocessed, unpasteurised milk from grass-fed cows.[31,61] If you look for such a farmer in your area you may be surprised to find one without too much difficulty.

Milk contains a sugar, called lactose. Some people get diagnosed as lactose intolerant. Well, after infancy we are all 'lactose intolerant' because the human gut does not produce an enzyme to digest lactose, called lactase.[37] So, how do many of us manage to digest milk? Because we have particular species of probiotic bacteria in the gut that do this work for us. Some of the most well-studied lactose-digesting species are physiological strains of E. coli.[38] People who cannot digest lactose have abnormal gut flora; they are lacking those probiotic bacteria. Instead of sentencing yourself to consuming highly processed lactose-free dairy products, you need to restore your gut flora by eating fermented foods and consuming good quality probiotics (read more on this subject in my GAPS book). Fermented dairy products, such as live yoghurt, kefir, natural traditional cheeses and butter have greatly reduced lactose contents and are usually tolerated well by lactose-intolerant people.[39] Pasteurisation of milk is a major contributor to lactose intolerance in the population. Raw fresh milk contains an active enzyme, lactase, to digest the lactose for you, but this enzyme is destroyed by pasteurisation. Many lactose-intolerant people find that they can digest raw milk perfectly well, while pasteurised milk causes all the usual unpleasant symptoms of lactose intolerance (bloating, indigestion, abdominal pain and diarrhoea).[34,36,37]

7. Buy unprocessed nuts and oily seeds.
Walnuts, almonds, brazil nuts, pecans, hazelnuts, cashew nuts, chestnuts, peanuts, sunflower seeds, pumpkin seeds, sesame seeds, etc. Do not buy them cooked, roasted, salted, coated or processed in any other way; buy them just shelled or in their shells. Nuts, sunflower, sesame and pumpkin seeds can be ground into flour consistency and used for making breads and

cakes at home. Nuts and seeds are full of good nutrients and are very important for us to eat. There is a mountain of research to show that regular consumption of these foods prevents heart disease, cancer, autoimmune disorders and many other health problems.[40,41,42,43]

It is not difficult to make nuts a normal part of your diet: just put a mixture of nuts, seeds and dried fruit into an attractive bowl and keep it on your coffee table in front of the TV set. You will be surprised how quickly your family gets used to snacking on these health-giving foods, instead of eating harmful, commercial processed snacks.

Keep in mind that nuts and seeds are very fibrous and can be difficult to digest. If you have digestive problems please study the GAPS Diet in my book *Gut And Psychology Syndrome*.[44]

8. Buy organic beans and pulses.
Buy them in their whole natural form and cook them at home. Avoid commercially available tinned beans and pulses, as they are processed foods full of sugar and other additives. Before cooking, all beans and pulses have to be pre-soaked in water for at least twelve hours to reduce the amounts of lectins and other harmful substances.[45,46] After soaking, rinse well under running water. Once cooked, they can be used in many recipes including bread and cakes. Avoid commercial flours made out of beans and pulses, as they have not been pre-soaked before grinding. There are many wonderful traditional recipes for cooking beans and pulses. However, if you have digestive problems, you may find them difficult to digest. For this reason many of the world's traditional cultures ferment their beans and

pulses, which makes them easy to digest, even for babies.[45]

9. Buy and use only natural fats.
We are talking about the fats that Mother Nature provided, and which traditional cultures around the world have been using for millennia: animal fats, fats on meats, butter and ghee, coconut and palm oil, *cold-pressed virgin* olive oil and other *cold-pressed virgin* natural oils (flax, hemp, avocado, evening primrose, walnut, sunflower, etc.).

Cold-pressed plant oils are difficult to produce and, therefore, are expensive. They are full of very fragile health-giving substances and must not be used for cooking as heat would destroy them. They are also easily damaged by oxygen and light, so we have to extract them with minimum exposure to air and keep them refrigerated in dark glass bottles.[47] Use these cold-pressed oils in small amounts as a dressing on ready served meals or take them as a supplement. They will provide you with essential fatty acids, antioxidants, vitamin E and many other good things. However, the majority of us don't have to buy these oils at all. Just eating fresh nuts, seeds (particularly sprouted), green leafy vegetables and other fresh vegetables, berries and fresh fruit will provide you with all the beneficial plant oils necessary.

Avoid all vegetable and cooking oils, widely available in supermarkets. They are extremely processed substances full of trans fats, solvents and other harmful chemicals. Consumption of these oils and margarines is one of the main causes of our many degenerative conditions.[53,54,55,56,57,58]

So, what fats do we use for cooking?

Cook with animal fats, such as lard, pork dripping, lamb fat, beef fat, goose fat, duck fat, etc. It is best to do what our grandmothers did: collect the fats yourself after cooking your meats; they will keep in a glass jar in your refrigerator for a long time and are excellent to use for cooking. Roasting a duck will provide you with a cup of excellent fat, which has been proven to be heart protective.[47,59] Roasting a large goose will provide you with even more of an excellent cooking fat. You can buy some of these fats from a traditional butcher. You can also cook with butter, ghee, natural coconut oil and palm oil. All these fats are healthy for us and very stable: they generally do not change their chemical structure when we cook with them, they can even be reused.[47]

I almost hear you asking a number of very common questions: "What about the 'deadly' saturated fats? Don't they cause heart disease, cancer and all other health problems? Aren't animal fats all saturated?"

These questions are the result of the relentless efforts made by the food industry to fight their competition. What is their competition? The natural fats, of course. There is not much profit to be made from the natural fats, while processed oils and fats bring very good profits.[53] So it is in the food industry's interest to convince everybody that natural fats are harmful for health, while their processed fats, hydrogenated and cooking oils are good for us.[55] We have been subjected to this propaganda for almost a century now; no wonder that many of us have succumbed to it.

The food industry singled out saturated fats in particular. How did that happen? The late Dr Mary Enig, an international expert in lipid biochemistry, explained: 'In the late 1950s, an American researcher Ancel Keys announced that the CHD epidemic was being caused by the hydrogenated vegetable fats; previously this same person had introduced the idea that saturated fat was the culprit. The edible oil industry quickly responded to this perceived threat to their products by mounting a public relations campaign to promote the belief that it was only the saturated fatty acid component in the hydrogenated oils that was causing the problem... From that time on, the edible fats and oils industry promoted the twin ideas that saturates (namely animal and dairy fats) were troublesome, and polyunsaturates (mainly corn oil and later soybean oil) were health-giving'.[47]

The wealthy food giants spend billions on employing an army of 'scientists' to provide them with 'scientific proof' of their claims. In the meantime the real science was, and is, providing us with the truth. However, it is the food giants who have the money to advertise their 'science' in all the popular media. Real science is too poor to spend money on that. As a result, the population hears only what the commercial powers want them to hear.

So, what is the truth? What does real science tell us?
1. Processed fats, hydrogenated fats and cooking vegetable oils cause atherosclerosis, heart disease and cancer.[55] This is a fact, proven overwhelmingly by real, honest science. All animal experiments to 'prove' the hypothesis that fats cause heart disease

were made with processed fats and processed oxidised cholesterol, which makes them completely invalid.[47,59]

2. Animal fats have nothing to do with heart disease, cancer or any other chronic illness; in fact they prevent them. Our human physiology needs these fats; they are important for us to eat on a daily basis.[59]

3. Saturated fats are heart protective: they lower levels of a harmful substance, called Lp(a), in the blood, reduce calcium deposition in the arteries and are the preferred source of energy for the heart muscle.[47] Saturated fats enhance our immune system, protect us from infections and are essential for the body to be able to utilise the unsaturated omega-3 and omega-6 fatty acids.[47,59] One of the most saturated fats that Nature has provided is coconut oil. It has been shown to be wonderfully healthy and therapeutic in most degenerative conditions.[47]

4. Animal fats contain a variety of different fatty acids, not just saturated ones.[60] Pork fat is 45% monounsaturated, 11% polyunsaturated and 44% saturated. Lamb fat is 38% monounsaturated, 2% polyunsaturated and 58% saturated. Beef fat is 47% monounsaturated, 4% polyunsaturated and 49% saturated. Butter is 30% monounsaturated, 4% polyunsaturated and 52% saturated. This is the natural composition of animal fats and our bodies use every bit, including the saturated part. If you want to understand how important every bit of the animal fat is for us, let us have a look at the composition of human breast

milk. The fat portion of the breast milk is 48% saturated, 33% monounsaturated and 16% polyunsaturated.[47,60] Our babies thrive beautifully on this
composition of fats, and the largest part of it is saturated.

5. We need all of the natural fats in natural foods, and
   saturated and monounsaturated fats need to be the
   largest part of our fat intake.

6. The simplistic idea that eating fat makes you fat is
   completely wrong. Consuming processed carbohydrates causes obesity.[48,49,60] Dietary fats go into the
   structure of your body: your brain, bones, muscles,
   immune system, etc. – every cell in the body is made
   out of fats to a large degree.[60]

These are the facts, which honest science has provided.
Unfortunately, most of us do not hear about the discov-
eries of honest science. Spreading any information in
this world costs money, which honest science doesn't
have. So, the population at large mostly gets information that serves somebody with a fat wallet. In order to
obtain the true information on any subject, we have to
search for it, rather than relying on the 'news' and
'scientific breakthroughs' unleashed on us by the popular media. This is particularly true for our understanding
of cholesterol.

What about cholesterol?

When we talk about animal fats, a question about
cholesterol invariably comes up, because everybody has
heard about cholesterol 'clogging up your arteries' and

'causing heart disease'. This idea came from the diet-heart hypothesis, first proposed in 1953.[59,61] Since then this hypothesis has been proven to be completely wrong by many scientific studies.[59,61] George Mann, eminent American physician and scientist, called the diet-heart hypothesis 'the greatest scientific deception of this century, perhaps of any century'.[62] Why? Because, while science was working on proving the hypothesis wrong, the medical, political and scientific establishments fully committed to it. To admit that they were wrong would do too much damage to their reputation, so they are not in a hurry to do that. In the meantime their closed ranks give complete freedom to the commercial companies to exploit the diet-heart hypothesis to their advantage.[59] Their relentless propaganda through the popular media ensures long life for the faulty diet-heart hypothesis.[59,61] Thanks to the promoters of the diet-heart hypothesis, everybody 'knows' that cholesterol is 'evil' and has to be fought at every turn. If you believe the popular media you would think that there is simply no level of cholesterol low enough.

The truth is that we humans cannot live without cholesterol. Let us see why?

Every cell of every organ in our bodies has cholesterol as a part of its structure. Cholesterol is an integral and very important part of our cell membranes; the membranes that make the cell wall and the walls of all organelles inside the cells.[63] And we are not talking about a few molecules of cholesterol here and there. In many cells, almost half of the cell wall is made from cholesterol.[63,64] Different kinds of cells in the body need different amounts of cholesterol, depending on their function and purpose.[65] The human brain is particularly rich in cholesterol: around 25% of all body cholesterol is taken by the brain.[66] Every cell and every structure in the brain and the rest of our nervous system needs cholesterol, not only to build itself but also to accomplish its many functions. The developing brain and eyes of the foetus and a newborn infant require large amounts of cholesterol.[66,68] If the foetus doesn't get enough cholesterol during development the child may be born with a congenital abnormality called a cyclopean eye.[67] Human breast milk provides a lot of cholesterol. Not only that, mother's milk provides a specific enzyme to allow the baby's digestive tract to absorb almost 100% of that cholesterol, because the developing brain and eyes of an infant require large amounts of it.[66] Children deprived of enough cholesterol in infancy end up with poor eyesight and brain function.[69] Manufacturers of infant formulas are aware of this fact, but following the anti-cholesterol dogma, they produce formulas with virtually no cholesterol in them.[66]

One of the most abundant materials in the brain and the rest of our nervous system is a fatty substance called myelin. Myelin coats every nerve cell and every nerve fibre like an insulating cover around electric wires.[70] Apart from insulation, it provides nourishment and protection for every tiny structure in our brain and the rest of the nervous system.[66] People who start losing their myelin develop a condition called multiple sclerosis. Well, 20% of myelin is cholesterol.[66] If you start interfering with the supply of cholesterol in the body, you put the very structure of the brain and the rest of the nervous system under threat. The synthesis of myelin in the brain is tightly connected with the synthesis of cholesterol.[71] People with multiple sclerosis and other neurological illnesses have antibodies against myelin. Due to these antibodies these patients have ongoing damage to the myelin in their brain and the rest of their nervous system. In order to rebuild myelin, their bodies require a lot of cholesterol. In my clinical experience, foods with high cholesterol and high animal fat content are an essential medicine for people with multiple sclerosis.

One of the most wonderful abilities we humans are blessed with is an ability to remember things – our human memory. How do we form memories? By our brain cells establishing connections with each other, called synapses. The more healthy synapses a person's brain can make, the more mentally able and intelligent that person is. Scientists have discovered that synapse formation is almost entirely dependent on cholesterol, which is produced by the brain cells in a form of apolipoprotein E.[72] Without the presence of this factor we could not form synapses, and hence we would not be able to learn or remember anything. Memory loss is one of the side effects of cholesterol-lowering medications, called statins. In my clinic I see growing numbers of people with memory loss who have been taking 'cholesterol pills'. Dr Duane Graveline, MD, former NASA scientist and astronaut, suffered such memory loss while taking his 'cholesterol pill'. He managed to save his memory by stopping the pill and eating lots of cholesterol-rich foods. Since then he has described his experience in his book *Lipitor – Thief of Memory, Statin*

Drugs and the Misguided War on Cholesterol.[73] Dietary cholesterol in fresh eggs, butter and other cholesterol-rich foods has been shown in scientific trials to improve memory in the elderly.[74,75] In my clinical experience, any person with memory loss or learning problems needs to have plenty of these foods every single day in order to recover.

Let us see which foods are rich in cholesterol.

1. Just like our own human brain, the brains of animals are rich in cholesterol. Animal brains are the richest food source for cholesterol, providing from 3100mg cholesterol (per 100g of beef brain) to 1352mg of cholesterol (per 100g of lamb brain).[76,77] In traditional cultures the brains of animals were considered to be a delicacy and were known to be very beneficial for health.

2. Organ meats are rich in cholesterol. Veal kidney can provide 791mg per 100g while chicken liver can provide 563mg per 100g. Other organ meats – livers and kidneys of other animals, heart, tongue, tripe, pancreas and poultry giblets will all provide good amounts of cholesterol. [74,75,77] Organ meats have always been considered to be health foods and sacred foods in traditional cultures all over the world.

3. Caviar (fish eggs) is the next richest source; it provides 588mg of cholesterol per 100g.[76,77]

4. Cod liver oil follows closely with 570mg of cholesterol per 100g. There is no doubt that the cholesterol element of cod liver oil plays an important role in all the well-known health benefits of this time-honoured health food.[75]

5. Fresh egg yolk takes the next place, with 424mg of cholesterol per 100g. I would like to repeat 'fresh egg yolk', not chemically mutilated egg powders (they contain chemically mutilated cholesterol)! [75,77]

6. Butter provides a good 218mg of cholesterol per 100g. We are talking about natural butter, not butter substitutes.[76]

7. Cold-water fish and shellfish, such as salmon, sardines, herring, mackerel and shrimps, provide good amounts of cholesterol, ranging from 173mg to 81mg per 100g. The proponents of low-cholesterol diets tell you to replace meats with fish. Obviously, they are not aware of the fact that fish can be almost twice as rich in cholesterol as meats.[76,77]

8. Lard provides 94mg of cholesterol per 100g. Other animal fats follow.[76,77]

These foods give the body a hand in supplying cholesterol, so it does not have to work as hard to produce its own. What a lot of people don't realise is that most cholesterol in the body does not come from food![74] The healthy human body produces cholesterol as it is needed. Cholesterol is such an essential part of our human physiology that the body has very efficient mechanisms to keep blood cholesterol at a certain level. When we eat more cholesterol, the body produces less; when we eat less cholesterol, the body produces more.[75] However, cholesterol-lowering drugs (statins) are a completely different matter. They interfere with the body's ability to produce cholesterol, and hence they do reduce the amount of cholesterol available for the body to use.[74,78] If we do not take cholesterol-lowering drugs, most of us don't have to worry about cholesterol. However, there are people whose bodies are unable to produce enough cholesterol due to toxicity and nutritional deficiencies.[61,74] Research shows that people who are unable to produce enough cholesterol are prone to emotional instability and behavioural problems. Low blood cholesterol has been routinely recorded in criminals who have committed murder and other violent crimes, people with aggressive and violent personalities, people prone to suicide and people with aggressive social behaviour and low self-control.[79,80,81] The late Oxford professor David Horrobin has stated: 'reducing cholesterol in the population on a large scale could lead to a general shift to more violent patterns of behaviour. Most of this increased violence would not result in death but in more aggression at work and in the family, more child abuse, more wife-beating and generally more unhappiness.'[79] People whose bodies are unable to produce enough cholesterol do need to have plenty of foods rich in cholesterol in order to provide their organs with this essential-to-life substance.

What else do our bodies need cholesterol for?

After the brain the organs hungriest for cholesterol are our endocrine glands: adrenals and sex glands. They produce steroid hormones. Steroid hormones in the body are made from cholesterol: testosterone, progesterone, pregnenolone, androsterone, oestrone, estradiol, corticosterone, aldosterone and others.[82,83] These hormones accomplish a myriad of functions in the body, from regulation of our metabolism, energy production, mineral assimilation, brain, muscle and bone formation to behaviour, emotions and reproduction. Our stressful modern lives consume a lot of these hormones, leading to a condition called 'adrenal exhaustion'. There are some herbal preparations on the market for adrenal exhaustion. However, the most important therapeutic measure is to provide your adrenal glands with plenty of dietary cholesterol.[84,85]

Cholesterol is essential for our immune system to function properly.[86,87,88,89] Animal experiments and human studies have demonstrated that immune cells rely on cholesterol in fighting infections and repairing themselves after the fight.[88,89] It has been recorded that people with high levels of cholesterol are protected from infections: they are four times less likely to contract AIDS,[90,92] they rarely get common colds,[93] and they recover from infections more quickly than people with 'normal' or low blood cholesterol.[91] On the other side of the spectrum, people with low blood cholesterol are prone to various infections, suffer from them longer and are more likely to die from an infection.[92] A diet rich in cholesterol has been demonstrated to improve these people's ability to recover from infections.[93] So, any person suffering from an acute or chronic infection needs to eat high-cholesterol foods to recover. Cod liver oil, one of the richest sources of cholesterol, has long been prized as the best remedy for the immune system. Those familiar with old medical literature will tell you that, until the discovery of antibiotics, a common cure for tuberculosis was a daily mixture of raw egg yolks and fresh cream (rich in cholesterol).[94] Our authorities are concerned about hospital infections, such as MRSA, which are getting more and more common. Almost every patient older than forty-five is put on statins in our hospitals, reducing their blood cholesterol and, as a result, impairing their immune function. There is no doubt that this common practice is a major cause of hospital infections!

It is beyond the scope of this book to talk about all the roles of cholesterol and animal fats in the human body. To understand this subject fully, please read my book *Put your heart in your mouth. What really causes heart disease and what we can do to prevent and even reverse it.*[95]

10. *Buy whole, unprocessed grains and prepare them properly before consuming!*

Buckwheat, millet, quinoa, oats, barley, brown rice, etc., to be cooked at home following traditional recipes. Do not buy processed grains or anything made out of flour. The most processed grains you can buy are breakfast cereals.

Whole grains should not be consumed without proper preparation, as they contain a number of harmful substances. They contain lectins, which can damage the gut wall and many other tissues and organs.[96,97] They contain phytates, which impair mineral absorption and can cause serious mineral deficiencies and bone loss; regular consumption of bran in particular is linked to osteoporosis.[98] They contain hard to digest proteins and starches. Wheat, rye, oats and barley contain a protein, called gluten, which is very difficult to digest for most of us and is positively dangerous for people with any digestive problems.[99,100] The popular advice to eat whole grains is misleading, because they are generally indigestible for humans and can do a lot of harm in the body. Herbivorous animals have several stomachs full of bacteria, which digest the plant matter for them.[101] We humans have only one stomach which, if it is healthy, has very little bacteria in it and has not been designed to digest grains without prior preparation. Traditional cultures around the world have known this fact for millennia and have always fermented or sprouted grains prior to cooking them. Fermentation reduces the amounts of lectins and phytates, predigests gluten and starch and releases nutrients.[102] To ferment, the grains can simply be soaked in water for several days; to speed up the process you can add a few spoonfuls of live yoghurt, kefir or whey to the water. When the grain has fermented, cook it in the usual way. Another excellent way to make grains more digestible is sprouting. Sprouting is a very easy procedure: soak unprocessed grains for 12–24 hours in water, then drain and keep moist in a warm place for a few days. As grains are seeds, they will sprout small shoots. In that form they are much more nourishing and easier to digest raw or cooked.

There is a very important point to make about grains, whether whole or not. Traditionally grains were always consumed with a good amount of natural fats: butter, ghee, olive oil, coconut or palm oil, goose fat, duck fat, pork fat, etc.[103,104] There is a lot of wisdom to that: grains are a concentrated source of carbohydrates and, unless their digestion is slowed down by fats, these carbohydrates will absorb quite quickly in the form of sugars, raising the blood sugar level too high, with many damaging consequences. So, the last thing you want to do is eat your grains fat free. The same goes for potatoes, sweet potatoes, yams, Jerusalem artichokes, parsnips and other starchy vegetables. They are a concentrated source of carbohydrates, so their digestion needs to be slowed down by adding good amounts of natural fats.

If you need to lose weight, suffer from diabetes or have digestive problems, avoid grains and starchy vegetables altogether (and, obviously, anything made out of them). People with any digestive problems must avoid all grains and starchy vegetables until their digestion improves.[105]

What about **bread**? The majority of people find it very difficult to avoid eating bread. People generally believe that bread is good for them because humankind has consumed it for thousands of years. The problem is that what we call bread nowadays is very different to what humans consumed even a hundred years ago! When did you last look at the ingredients list of the bread you buy? You will find that most breads on the shelves of our supermarkets and our bakeries are extremely processed products, full of dozens of chemicals, soy protein isolate, margarine, harmful vegetable oils, modified starch, hydrogenated oils, etc., etc. Bread is probably the biggest source of processed foods that the majority of us eat today.

If you want bread, make your own, following traditional time-proven bread making recipes. These are not the recipes that come with your bread making machine! I highly recommend a wonderful recipe book by Sally Fallon, *Nourishing Traditions*, which will provide you with traditional recipes from different cultures of the world.[104] If you live in an area where your local baker makes traditional sourdough bread, then consider yourself extremely lucky.

Remember, that if you need to lose weight, suffer from diabetes or have digestive problems, avoid grains and starchy vegetables altogether and anything made out of them. Bread made out of grains (generally wheat or rye flour) will do you no favours. However, if you bake bread using nuts and oily seeds, ground into flour consistency, you will do your body a lot of good. You can buy almond flour (ground almonds) and coconut flour commercially or grind nuts, sunflower and pumpkin seeds into a flour consistency. Add some eggs and butter, mix and bake and you will have a delicious bread or a basis for making a cake.

11. What about sweet taste?
Nature has provided us with excellent sweeteners: natural, unprocessed honey and dried fruit (make sure the fruit is natural, not coated in sugar, syrup or anything else). These sweet things are full of life-giving nutrients and do not damage the body.[104,105,107] Avoid sugar and all artificial sweeteners. If you want to bake a cake, dried fruit such as dates, figs and raisins will sweeten it for you beautifully and make your cake more nutritious.

Before the introduction of sugar in the 17th century honey and fruit were the only sweeteners that humans used in their diet. Starting from the end of the 17th century, sugar, being cheaper and more available, replaced honey in people's diet, beginning an era of sugar-related health problems. Honey is natural to our physiology, and far from damaging our health it has a lot of health-giving properties. Honey has been used as food and medicine for thousands of years. In Greek mythology honey was considered a 'food fit for the gods'. There are dozens of books written about the health-giving properties of natural honey.[107] It works as an antiseptic and provides vitamins, minerals, amino acids and many other bioactive substances.[107,108,109] Depending on the variety of flowers from which a particular honey has been collected, different flavours and compositions of nutrients and bio-active substances can be found in the honey. Traditionally honey has been used to treat digestive disorders, chest and throat infections, arthritis, anaemia, insomnia, headaches, debility and cancer.[107,108,111,112,113,114] It can be applied therapeutically to open wounds, eczema patches, skin rashes, skin and mouth ulcers and erosions.[106,107,108,109,110]

Dried fruit will provide you with all the vitamins, minerals and other beneficial substances that fruit contains, but in concentrated amounts. As a result, in every traditional culture of the world dried fruit was used as medicine for various health problems. It was specifically given to pregnant women and to couples who were trying to conceive a baby; to people with tuberculosis and other chronic infections; to people with neurological and psychological symptoms and to people recovering from severe illness.[115,116,117,118,119] Regular consumption of dried dates, raisins, figs, currants, berries, prunes, etc. will do much more for your health than the most expensive supplements in the world. Apart from that, they are the natural sweets Mother Nature gave us. So, instead of buying commercial sweets, which damage your children's health, teach them to eat dried fruit.

12. Eat fermented foods, prepared according to traditional methods.

Fermentation is the use of beneficial microbes to preserve food for long periods of time. We have already mentioned natural live yoghurt, kefir and cheese – these are fermented foods. Sauerkraut (fermented cabbage), kimchi and other fermented vegetables will provide you with wonderful nutrition and beneficial bacteria. Good quality wine, natural kvass and natural beer without additives are fermented drinks and are good for us in moderate amounts.

Traditionally every culture of the world made fermented foods: people fermented dairy, grains, meats, fish, beans, pulses, vegetables and fruit because that was the only way they could preserve food for a long time.[120] Foods used to be seasonal and there were no supermarkets where one could buy anything all year round. For example, when your cabbages were ready you had to do something with them, or they would rot away and you would be left without cabbage for the rest of the year. So people made sauerkraut and consumed it until the next harvest, taking in mouthfuls of beneficial probiotic bacteria, active enzymes and other wonderful substances that only a fermented food would provide.[104,120] The process of fermentation predigests the food and releases its nutrients, which makes them more accessible for our bodies to use. For example, sauerkraut has almost 20 times more bio-available vitamin C in it than the same amount of fresh cabbage.[104] The famous British explorer James Cook, who discovered Australia and New Zealand, had barrels of sauerkraut on his ships to prevent scurvy in his crew.[103,104] Through the ages our physiology became used to having fermented food on a daily basis; it has become essential for us to stay healthy. Since we invented refrigeration, we humans have almost stopped consuming these foods. As a result, we are depriving ourselves of all the wonderful benefits that fermented foods would provide: probiotic bacteria to keep our gut flora healthy, easy-to-digest nutrients, active enzymes to keep us young and energetic and many other good things.

There are many easy fermentation recipes that you can use at home. You can find these recipes online and in many good books on nutrition.

13. Drink freshly pressed fruit and vegetable juices.
You will need to have a good juicer at home and get fresh, organic fruit and vegetables to juice. It is important to use organic produce, because if you juice non-organic fruit and vegetables you will get concentrated amounts of pesticides and other agricultural chemicals in your glass of juice. Thousands of people all over the world have freed themselves from the most deadly diseases with juicing; dozens of books have been published on this subject, full of testimonies and wonderful recipes.[121,122] Some very big names in natural medicine have strongly advocated juicing and used it actively in the treatment of their patients – people like Dr Max Gerson and Dr Norman Walker for example. Hundreds of scientific studies have been published on the health benefits of fresh raw fruit and vegetables. Juices provide all the goodness from these fruit and vegetables in a concentrated form and in large amounts. For example, to make a glass of carrot juice you need a pound of carrots. Nobody can eat a pound

of carrots at once, but you can get all the nutrition from them by drinking the juice. The digestive system has virtually no work to do when digesting freshly pressed juice; they get absorbed in 20–25 minutes, providing the body with a concentrated amount of nutrients. With juicing you can consume large quantities of fresh vegetables and fruit every day in the most digestible and pleasant form.

Many children in our modern world will not eat fruit and vegetables, and I know quite a few adults like that as well. Juices, being so tasty, can provide an excellent solution to this problem. Drinking freshly extracted juice will provide you and your child with many essential vitamins, minerals and other useful nutrients.[123,124] A combination of pineapple, carrot and a little bit of beetroot in the morning will prepare the digestive system for the coming meals, stimulate stomach acid production and pancreatic enzymes production. A mixture of carrot, apple, celery and beetroot has a wonderful liver-cleansing ability. Green juices from leafy vegetables (spinach, lettuce, coriander, parsley, dill, carrot and beet tops) with some tomato and lemon are a great source of magnesium and iron and help your body to remove toxic metals. Cabbage, apple and celery juice stimulates digestive enzyme production and is a great kidney cleanser. There is an endless number of healthy and tasty variations you can make from whatever organic fruit and vegetables you have available at home.[123,124,125] To make the juice taste nice, particularly for children, generally try to have 50% of less tasty but highly therapeutic ingredients – carrot, small amount of beetroot (no more than 5% of the juice mixture), celery, cabbage, lettuce, greens (such as spinach, parsley, dill, basil, fresh nettle leaves, beet tops and carrot tops) – and 50% of some tasty ingredients: pineapple, apple, orange, grapefruit, grapes, mango, etc.

Any person with a degenerative disease, any person under a lot of stress, any person recovering from jet-lag or from an infection, and any person who is run down or simply tired would benefit tremendously from drinking freshly pressed juices.[88,89]

What about fibre? Drinking juices doesn't mean that you stop eating fresh fruit and vegetables. You should carry on eating fruit and vegetables as usual. Treat the juices like a supplement of concentrated nutrients in a glass. They should be taken on an empty stomach 20–25 minutes before food and 2–2½ hours after a meal. Freshly pressed juices are highly perishable; they need to be consumed within a few minutes from extracting (30 minutes maximum). So, make just enough to be consumed immediately. Whatever has not been consumed can be frozen as ice lollies for children or ice cubes for making cold drinks later. Children, in particular, love freshly pressed juices. You can make smoothies from them by mixing the juice with mashed avocado or banana and adding it to yoghurt or home-made ice cream and sorbet.

But can't we just buy juices from shops? The answer is a big NO! Juices in the shops have been processed and pasteurised, which destroys all the enzymes and most vitamins and phytonutrients. They are a source of processed sugar, which will feed abnormal bacteria and fungi in the gut and upset your blood sugar level.[125] In freshly extracted juice the natural sugars are balanced with active enzymes, minerals, and other nutrients, which turn them into nourishment and energy for the body. When you make your juice at home you know what you put into it, you know that it is fresh without any contamination or oxidation, and you can have great fun mixing different fruit and vegetables together to make different tasty combinations. There is a large number of books written on juicing with wonderful recipes for every health problem and every occasion.[121,122]

14. Beverages.
We have already mentioned fermented beverages, such as good-quality wine and home-made kvass. We have also discussed freshly pressed juices. All these beverages are good for us in reasonable amounts.

Apart from those it is important to drink plenty of water. What kind of water? As natural and as clean as possible and that, unfortunately, does not include tap water in many parts of the world. Tap water contains many additives, which will absorb into your bloodstream and cause damage: chlorine, fluoride, nitrates and agricultural chemicals to mention a few. That is why it is important to filter your tap water.

A lot of bottled water on the market is no better than your tap water. When buying bottled water, look for natural mineral water from an established and known producer, preferably in a glass bottle as plastic leaches harmful chemicals into the water.[126,127,128,129,130] Lucky are those people who live near a clean well or a spring, where they can drink natural water without anything added to it. It is a good idea to add a slice of lemon or a teaspoon of organic apple cider vinegar to your glass of water, as they will add alkalising minerals and other good qualities.

Many of us like to have a hot beverage, such as tea or coffee. These drinks are stimulants and a lot of people get addicted to them without knowing it. The way to find out if you are addicted is to stop drinking coffee and tea for a few days. An addicted person will get serious headaches and cravings for these beverages. If you are not addicted to them, there is nothing wrong with having a cup of tea or a cup of coffee occasionally. But make sure that you have good-quality tea and coffee, freshly made out of quality organic ingredients, not instant and not processed.[131]

What you also have to understand is that coffee and tea are dehydrating for your body. This means that they make your body acid and very thirsty for water. Make sure that you rehydrate yourself with plenty of water and juicy fruit and vegetables at other times of the day. It will also help if you have your tea with a slice of lemon instead of milk and eat a good piece of juicy fruit with your cup of coffee. Replace sugar with honey and, if you want a snack with your hot drink, a helping of natural nuts and dried fruit will remove many of the negative influences that coffee or tea may have on your body. Cheese and honey also make a good snack to have with your cup of tea or coffee. Make sure that the cheese is natural and made according to traditional practices. It goes without saying that you should avoid eating biscuits and cakes with your hot beverage, which unfortunately is exactly what people commonly serve.

There are many herbal teas on the market and their variety is growing. Most herbs are medicinal, which means that they will have a particular effect on your physiology. That is why many of them do not suit everybody. If you find an herbal tea that suits you, then make sure that it is organic, as non-organic herbal teas may contain toxic metals and other contaminants.[132,133]

It goes without saying that you must avoid all pop drinks and soft beverages, including cordials, if you want to avoid chronic disease. They are made out of sugar and chemicals – a double toxic attack on your body.[134,135] The 'sugar-free' soft drinks are even worse: they contain artificial sweeteners, which can be even more toxic than sugar.[136,137]

Strong alcoholic beverages are something you may want to indulge in very occasionally and in very small amounts. They load your liver with a lot of work, making it unable to handle the other toxins floating in your blood, which leaves them free to cause damage. Excessive alcohol and its toxic by-products also directly cause many health problems.[138]

We have already talked about beer. Here I would like to add that it is made from grains and, in the process of fermentation, the starch from grain is broken down into various forms of sugars. Beer is a concentrated source of processed carbohydrates – a syrup, which is made out of sugars that don't taste sweet (many sugars in Nature taste bland or even bitter). These sugars absorb quickly into your bloodstream and can cause high blood sugar level and high insulin level. Both are dangerous, as they lay the ground for excessive weight gain, diabetes and heart disease.[139] If you already have a predisposition to any of these health problems, it is a good idea to reduce your beer consumption or to avoid it altogether.

In conclusion

When feeding yourself or your family please remember these simple rules: never economise on food and never compromise when it comes to food! Because if you do not eat well, you will not be healthy, and if you do not have your health, you will have no life.

Compromise and economise on clothes, cars, entertainment, toys, etc., etc., but never on food. Buy good quality and fresh food. Organic is better than non-organic. Local produce is better than exotic food that has had to travel half across the world. Fruit and vegetables, grown in a private garden, are better than fruit and vegetables from any supermarket. Pasture-fed animals are better than those raised on grains or commercial animal foods. Traditionally grown and prepared food is better than modern inventions. Pick your own berries, fruit and vegetables whenever you have a chance. Prepare your food with love and care, do not burn or overcook it. Use traditional cooking methods, do not use microwave ovens. Those of you who make these simple changes will gain endless benefits.

Have you ever wondered what a 'balanced meal' means? Our mainstream will tell you that it is proportions of carbs to protein and fat. No, that is not what it means! It means that all your taste buds are singing praises to the meal you eat. Our taste buds are specialised: some perceive sweet, some sour, some perceive salty, some astringent, some perceive pungent and some perceive bitter. All of these tastes should be present in the meal. So, when you make a meal, add some sweet vegetables (carrots and beets for example), some bitter (celery leaves, dark-green leaves, aubergines, courgette, spices and herbs), some chillies, garlic, onion or herbs for a pungent taste, some natural salt or seaweed, broccoli, cauliflower, asparagus and turnip for an astringent taste, and some fermented vegetables, vinegar or lemon to satisfy the sour taste. These guidelines will produce very tasty and satisfying meals for you. They have been an important part of Ayurveda – the full-of-wisdom ancient traditional medicine in India.[140] But of course the most important parts of any meal are the meat and the fat! We can cook our vegetables without meat, but we must add good amounts of fat into it! It is the fat that will bring out all the tastes and extract beneficial nutrients from the vegetables. The best fat to cook your vegetables with comes from animals: bacon fat, pork dripping, lard, tallow, lamb fat, goose fat, butter and ghee. Fat is essential for our bodies to be able to use minerals, vitamins, protein and many other nutrients. The more animal fat you add to your meal the more nourishment your body will get out of it.

Eating out a lot is a very unhealthy habit (that includes takeaway meals), because you have no idea what kind of ingredients and cooking methods were used to make your meal. And you have no idea *who* cooked your meal and with what attitude.

Why is the attitude of the cook important? It is very important because cooking is alchemy. The most important part of any alchemy is the alchemist: the person who makes the meal. The most important actions of the alchemist in the process are his thoughts and attitudes – this is what creates the magic. We, humans, are powerful creatures! If a person who cooks your meal doesn't like you and wishes you ill, this energy will permeate the meal they prepare for you. This meal will not bring you good health! The meals you eat must be produced by people who love you, who wish you to have the best health and happiness. This kind of meal will bring you good health and healing from any illness. The attitude of the cook is vital! If you don't have somebody loving to cook your meals for you, then cook them yourself and do it with love. When cooking, don't allow yourself to think about anything that makes you angry, resentful or negative. The meals cooked with these attitudes will not digest well and will not bring you good health, no matter how good the ingredients and the recipe may be.

The person who cooks for the family holds the health of that family in her or his hands. This is power! The health of any nation is not in the hands of governments or the medical profession. It is in the hands of those who cook for that nation! If the nation consumes things cooked by some faceless factories, then that nation will have poor health – exactly what is happening in Western countries. In traditional societies women knew the value of food; they knew that there is nothing more powerful in its effect on human health than food. They knew that, through cooking, they were holding the health of their families in their hands. They would never relinquish that power to anyone else! Women knew what foods to use for what occasions: what is good for babies, what is good for pregnant women, what is good for a couple trying to conceive a baby, what is good for any illness or injury, and what is good for the elderly to eat. Women knew the herbs growing in their location and used them extensively in cooking. This sacred knowledge was passed through generations: from mother to daughter and from grandmother to granddaughter. From the dawn of the food industry, women started losing this knowledge. The food industry advertising lured them away from cooking and deceived them into relinquishing their God-given power – to hold the health of their loved ones in their own hands! The result is the misery of sickness in Western families, which is getting deeper with every generation.

To support their commercial aims the industry has pronounced cooking as 'dirty' and 'beneath' women. Unfortunately, many women have succumbed to this propaganda, thinking that they gain some ill-conceived 'equality' with men. There is no 'equality' in Nature; instead there is beauty of diversity and difference! Nature celebrates difference and unity of opposites complementing each other. Imagine if day decided to be 'equal' with night? Or winter decided to be 'equal' with summer? There is a glorious difference between women and men; they have different functions to fulfil in Nature. Men's physiology represents moving forward, discovering and opening new horizons and possibilities, which in the history of humanity often led to wars and destruction. Women's physiology represents nurture, care, healing and repair. Women give birth to children;

and bringing up children requires peace and prosperity. That is why more often than not in human history it is women who brought peace to their countries, directly or through influencing their men. So, from Nature's point of view, it is a woman's role to nurture her family! Women in the West must reclaim their power to look after the health of their families through food. Women who have done that are truly happy and fulfilled. And, in our modern world, it is possible to do that and hold a profession as well. Of course, there are always exceptions to any rule: in some families men are more nurturing than women, and they do the cooking. Whoever is in charge of feeding the family must be a person who loves that family, and who understands the responsibility they take upon themselves – holding the health of their loved ones in their hands.

Cooking is not difficult. Following the guidelines in this book, anyone can become a good cook! Forget the recipe books. Cooking is a very creative activity, enjoy it and create your own unique meals every time you cook. Just keep in mind: you are cooking for good health (not convenience, not expediency or anything else). Do your shopping and cooking with this thought. As a result you will lay a solid foundation for your own health and the health of your family. And a healthy family is usually a happy family! And if your family consists of only one person – you, then make meals for this small family with as much love as you would have for a large family.

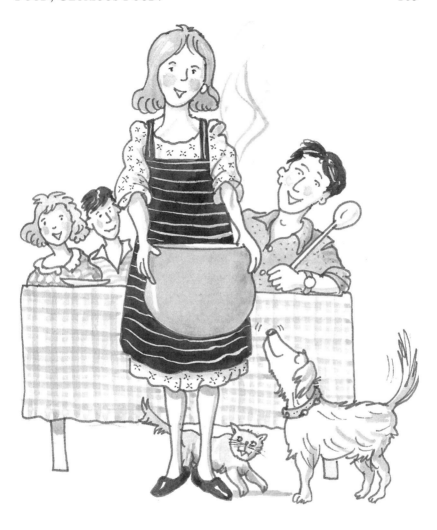

Fasting

We live in a polluted world, and a lot of this pollution gets stored in our bodies.[1,2,3,4,5,7,9] On top of that we add toxic substances to our bodies in the form of processed foods, personal care products, environmental pollution, pharmaceutical medications, agricultural chemicals, electromagnetic pollution, radiation and other man-made things.[1,2,3,4,6,7,8,9] This man-made toxicity leads to the development of many chronic diseases and, ultimately, cancer.[3,4] So it is important to cleanse. Consuming natural fresh foods, where whole, full-fat animal products (the *Feeding Foods*) are combined with fresh organic plant foods (the *Cleansing Foods*), will prevent many diseases. However, eating properly for some people may not be enough in our modern world, full of man-made pollution.[1,7] That is why it is a good idea for many of us to have periods of cleansing, even those who consider themselves to be fairly healthy.[7]

Fasting is one of the oldest and most effective ways of cleaning your body on the inside.[10,11] Our bodies spend large amounts of energy on digesting and metabolising food on a daily basis. When we stop eating or reduce it dramatically, the body re-directs its energy to other jobs, such as removing toxins and parasites, and healing itself.[11] Fasting has an excellent record of curing all sorts of 'incurable' conditions –from rheumatoid arthritis to cancer.[10,11,12] In people without serious illness regular fasting will clean and rejuvenate the body and prevent disease.

What is fasting?

FASTING IS AVOIDANCE OF ALL FEEDING / BUILD-ING FOODS – ANIMAL FOODS (MEAT, FISH, EGGS AND DAIRY).

On a fast we can eat all the *Cleansing Foods* – plant foods, available to us, we can choose a few plant foods and avoid the rest, or we can remove all food completely.

There are a number of forms of fasting to choose from. Let us have a look at them, starting from the most difficult and restrictive ones. But before we start it is important to emphasise that *pregnant women and small children must not fast. People who are malnourished and have low body weight also must not fast.*

Water fasting is complete abstinence from food; the person drinks water and consumes nothing else.[10,11] It is one of the oldest and very effective ways to cleanse and rejuvenate your body. Many religions advocate regular water fasting.[13] No matter how short or long you make your water fast, you will derive benefits from it. You can fast at home one day a week, or three days at a time every few months, or just miss an evening meal a couple of times per week. But if you want to attempt a longer water fast (more than three days) of one week, two weeks, three weeks (some people fast as long as 45 days), it is essential to do so under professional supervision. There are many nuances to a long water fast, and it is easy to get into trouble if you are not experienced. Coming out of a long water fast is also quite a special procedure and needs professional supervision. There are some well-established fasting clinics around the word.[14] It is expensive to go to a clinic, but if you have never fasted in your life and would like to do a long fast, it is worth doing so. Having done the first fast under supervision, you will have gained experience and may be able to fast again without supervision.

In many people's minds fasting is associated with vegetarianism. Indeed, quite a few books on fasting finish off with an author's ardent attempt to turn the reader into a vegetarian or a vegan. Unfortunately, that pushes people away from the whole idea of fasting. Let's be absolutely clear about this: fasting has nothing to do with vegetarianism or veganism! No matter what your dietary persuasion is you can benefit from the healing and rejuvenating properties of water fasting. Many books on fasting tell you to come out of water fasting on plant foods only. Again, this is nothing but an attempt to turn the reader into a vegetarian. Coming out of water fasting should be done by slow introduction of both animal foods and plants. For a detailed explanation on how to come out from any fast please look at the end of this chapter.

Juice fasting. A juice fast is when the person consumes only freshly pressed fruit and vegetable juices (including green juices), as well as water.[12,15] It is often called a 'juice feast' as the person can drink unlimited amounts of freshly pressed delicious juices (usually 12 glasses a day!). The juices should contain no fibre, so they have to be strained well. Unfortunately, during juice fasting large amounts of plant sugars are consumed with the juices, so this approach can be a problem for people with unstable blood sugar, candida overgrowth, diabetes and other sugar-sensitive health problems. There are a number of well-written books on juice fasting with detailed explanations and testimonies.[12,15]

Liquitarianism is another form of fasting. It refers to avoidance of all food apart from clear liquids: herbal teas, vegetable broth, miso soup, rice milk, nut milk (made from almonds, coconut, sunflower seeds, etc.), freshly pressed juices, green drinks (such as spirulina and chlorella), rice water and other clear liquids, including water. Many health benefits have been reported by people using this form of fasting.[13,15] I would recommend adding bone broth and meat stock to this form of fasting, particularly for people with digestive problems. While your gut is resting on the fast, the meat stock and bone broth will provide substances that will heal and repair your digestive wall.

Fruit fasting. On a fruit fast the person eats only raw organic fruit of their choice; a mixture of seasonal juicy fruit is recommended. Chewing the fruit thoroughly is very important to reduce the sugar content (which is digested by enzymes in your saliva) and to break apart the fibre.[16] This fast can only be attempted when there is an ample supply of fresh organic fruit from your own orchard or somebody else's organic orchard nearby. Fruit must ripen on the tree, so it must be local. It is not a good idea to try this fast on fruit bought in a supermarket. Even labelled organic, commercial fruit is likely to have been grown on exhausted soils and picked unripe.

Mono diets. On mono diets people eat only one food and nothing else for a period of time. Examples of these are brown-rice mono diet, milk-only diet, grapes-only diet, apples-only diet, etc. The idea of a mono diet was proposed by a German health educator and fasting enthusiast Arhold Ehret in the early 1900s.[17] It was popularised by a South African political activist Johanna Brandt in the 1920s, who claimed to have cured herself from stomach cancer by eating only grapes for some 40 days. She wrote a book about it called *The Grape Cure*.[18]

Veganism (eating only plants) is a form of fasting. It is essential that all the plants are organic and in their natural form, preferably cooked at home. The plants provide a huge amount of cleansing substances for the body to use, particularly when they are consumed raw, sprouted or fermented.[19] Cooked plants, particularly starchy plants, provide a lot of glucose for the body to process. The body can use a limited amount of glucose for producing energy. If glucose comes in excess the body converts it into fat and stores it in the fat tissues.[20] Plants provide a lot of fibre and indigestible starch, which feed the gut flora in the bowel.[21] If the person has a damaged gut flora dominated by pathogens, this can create a lot of gas production, abnormal stools and abdominal discomfort. Plants are unable to provide enough protein or fat suitable for building the human body or sustaining its physical structure.[22,23,24] That is why veganism must not be followed for long periods of time, and must never be imposed on pregnant women, babies, growing children or malnourished people with low body mass.[25,26,27,28,29,30,31]

There are several varieties of a vegan fast. Some people eat all the plants available to them: grains (including bread), beans and pulses, vegetables, fruit, nuts and vegetable oils. Other people avoid grains, particularly people with gluten intolerances and digestive problems. Every person designs his or her diet depending on individual tolerance and preferences. Availability of organic fresh produce is a big factor in designing your vegan fast. All processed foods and drinks, made with flour, sugar, soy, vegetable oils and chemical additives must be avoided. Otherwise there will be no cleansing, but more pollution coming into the body. It is essential to listen to your body and introduce animal foods when you get a desire for them. This desire is the signal from your body that it has finished cleansing and wants to be fed. People who follow veganism for emotional or spiritual reasons often don't listen to their bodies and miss that point, which leads to serious nutritional deficiencies and

health problems.[30,31,32] This is what happened to
Helen. Remember those Hindu pilgrims? They follow a
vegan fast for a maximum of 41 days. For the majority
of people just a few days or a couple of weeks is usually
enough, maximum two months!

How to come out from a long fast

During fasting, the production of digestive enzymes is
reduced dramatically, so we cannot suddenly fill our
stomachs with lots of food, because we will not be able
to digest it. We need food that is easy to digest, and we
need to introduce it slowly and gradually, starting with
small amounts. As the body has not been fed for a
while, we need to introduce *feeding foods* straight away
– meats, fish, eggs and dairy. It is best to introduce food
in its raw state, because raw fresh food is equipped with
active enzymes to assist your digestive system in breaking this food down.[33] We need to consume raw animal
foods in combination with herbs, raw honey and
freshly squeezed lemon juice, which also have many
enzymes to assist digestion.[34] We should add natural
salt and black pepper to the meals to stimulate stomach
acid production.[33,34] We can have some raw vegetables
with our animal foods to add some fibre and variety. We
can have some raw fruit and nuts between meals as
snacks (as long as the person is not prone to flatulence,
belching or reflux). The only cooked food we should
consume, when coming out of a long fast, is meat stock.
Freshly made meat stock is soothing and healing for the
gut lining, it will help your digestive system to recover
from the fast quickly and fully.

Let us have a look at what to eat day by day.

Day 1 after the fast

- Start your day with a cup of hot meat stock. Chicken stock is the best. To make it put a whole chicken, including the feet and some giblets, into a 6-litre pan, add a tablespoon of natural salt and fill the pan with water. Bring to the boil, then reduce the heat to a simmer, cover and cook for 2 hours. When ready, strain the stock into another pan, cool it down and keep in a refrigerator. The cooked chicken from the stock should be consumed by somebody else; your gut is not ready for it after a long fast. Add a tablespoon of live yoghurt or kefir into every cup of the meat stock you drink, to provide probiotic microbes. In order not to kill these beneficial microbes, make sure that the stock is not too hot when adding the yoghurt or kefir.
- Before putting the chicken into the pot for making the stock, cut out one breast from it leaving the skin on the chicken (the skin should be cooked in the stock). Do not make the breast wet. If you washed it, then dry it well. Cut the breast into bite-size pieces, squeeze half a lemon onto it, add half a teaspoon of honey, some freshly ground black pepper and natural salt, a tablespoon of homemade raw organic yoghurt or kefir, a few cloves of fresh garlic, chopped finely, some chopped parsley or dill and olive oil. If you have some fermented vegetables, you can add a tablespoon of sauerkraut, kimchi, fermented carrots, fermented cucumbers or any other home-fermented vegetables.

Mix all the ingredients well, cover the dish and leave to marinade at room temperature (if it is not too hot) or in the fridge for 2 hours. This is your lunch and dinner. You can have it with a small salad made from organic lettuce, onion, tomato and cucumber; use lemon juice, natural salt and olive oil as dressing. Try not to eat all of it at once, eat half at lunch and another half at dinner. Chew your food very well in order to make it more digestible.

- In the evening drink another cup of the meat stock you made. Don't forget to add some kefir or yoghurt to the stock.
- Drink some water between meals and freshly made herbal teas. The teas should be made from loose fresh or dried herbs, not from tea bags. Fresh mint and lavender leaves, willow leaves and small branches, ginger root and other herbs will make a refreshing tea.
- Before bed put a cup of organic shelled sunflower seeds into a glass jar and cover the seeds with water. They will soak overnight and become crunchy and easy to digest. In the morning drain the water, cover the jar with a clean cloth and leave the seeds to sprout. You can have a teaspoon of these seeds tomorrow with your lunch.

Day 2 after the fast

- Start your day with a cup of hot meat stock (yesterday's meat stock is fine) with a raw egg mixed into it (both the white and the yolk). Make sure to buy eggs that come from pastured organic chickens. In about an hour have another cup of meat stock with a raw egg in it. Don't forget to add some kefir or yoghurt to the stock.

- Made the same marinade as yesterday, but with raw lamb or beef this time. The meat needs to be fresh and dry (no added water). Eat a small portion for lunch and a small portion for dinner. You can have it with some ripe avocado, a teaspoon of your soaked sunflower seeds and a small salad.
- In the evening drink another cup of the meat stock you made. Don't forget to add some kefir or yoghurt. You can add another fresh egg to the stock.

Day 3 after the fast

- For breakfast you can have two soft-boiled eggs and a cup of hot meat stock with some kefir or yoghurt in it. Eat a good amount of raw organic butter with your eggs: for every mouthful of egg add a mouthful of butter and chew them together. The stock, which you made on the first day, will still be fresh enough for you to consume today, as long as it has been kept in the fridge.
- For lunch make the same marinade with any fresh meat or fish you have. Eat some ripe avocado and a salad with it. Add two tablespoons of sprouted sunflower seeds to your salad.
- In the afternoon have some herbal tea. You can have a little honey with it, some fruit and a few raw nuts.
- In the evening drink another cup of meat stock. Don't forget to add some kefir or yoghurt. You can add 1–2 fresh raw eggs to the stock.

Day 4 after the fast

- You can start your day with soft-boiled eggs and butter again, as yesterday. You can have a small salad and add to it the rest of your sprouted sunflower seeds. You can have a cup of herbal tea and eat some raw cheese and honey.
- Today you will need to make fresh meat stock. You can make it from lamb, pork, beef or fish. You need bones, joints, skin, a bit of meat and offcuts to make good stock. Add water, salt and freshly crushed black pepper corns and cook for 2–3 hours. If you want to make a fish stock, you will need to fill half of the pan with fresh small fish or with skins, heads and bones of larger fish. Fish stock can be cooked for one hour. Strain the hot stock into a clean dry pan, cool and keep in the fridge. Take some of this stock and make a soup: add chopped vegetables (carrot, onion, cabbage, celery, courgette or any other available vegetables) and cook for 25–30 minutes. While the soup is cooking, take all the soft tissues off the bones and joints (which you made the stock with) and chop them into bite-size pieces. Extract the bone marrow from tubular bones (bang the cooked bone on a thick wooden chopping board and the bone marrow will fall out). When the soup is ready add the meats and bone marrow to the soup together with some chopped garlic and parsley or dill. Enjoy this soup with some sour cream, kefir, or yoghurt.
- In the afternoon have some herbal tea. You can have a little honey with it and some raw high-fat cheese.

- In the evening drink another cup of meat stock. Don't forget to add some kefir or yoghurt. You can add 1–2 fresh raw eggs to the stock.

In the following days you can gradually introduce cooked meats, fish and eggs, and all other foods. Avoid grains, beans and lentils for a few days; they are difficult to digest. Allow your digestive system to adjust to food and start producing normal amounts of digestive enzymes before introducing these plant foods. Avoid all processed foods! Only food, made at home from fresh natural ingredients, should be consumed.

The animal foods, you have introduced after your fast, will stimulate production of your own digestive enzymes. These enzymes are proteins. Animal foods will provide your body with plenty of building materials to make these enzymes from.[33] Some people are concerned about eating raw meat because of fear of infections. There is no need to fear this if the meat is fresh and local, particularly if it is organic and pasture-fed. Avoid raw pork, but fresh beef, lamb, organic chicken and game can be eaten raw. Fresh meat has many active enzymes that protect it from microbes.[34,35] Apart from that, the marinade that you add to the meat will remove any possibility of infection. Lemon juice, garlic, olive oil, salt and black pepper are known to have antimicrobial properties.[36,37] If you add some fermented vegetables (or/and homemade raw yoghurt or kefir) they will provide probiotic (beneficial) microbes, which will not allow any pathogenic ones to develop in the food.[38] Raw meat stimulates stomach acid production, which is a powerful antiseptic. A healthy stomach at the beginning of a meal can produce enough acid to have pH 1–2, which kills most microbes in existence.[39] Eating fresh raw meat is perfectly safe and will provide many benefits: unadulterated protein, fats, enzymes, vitamins and minerals – all in the most digestible form for the human body. When we cook meat we change its structure, altering the structure of proteins, destroying enzymes and many vitamins and reducing its nutritional value.[33,34,35] People have recovered from many chronic illnesses by eating raw meat, raw eggs and raw dairy.[35]

Traditional cultures around the world ate raw meat, raw fish, raw eggs and raw milk products for millennia. There are written accounts of how native American people ate their meat raw. When Europeans came to America they forced the natives to start cooking their meat.[40] Eskimos and other people of the far North consumed most of their fish and meat raw: fresh, dried or fermented.[41] These traditions still remain in some of our modern recipes: gravlax in Sweden, stake tartar in France, beef carpaccio and carne cruda in Italy, sashimi in Japan, yookhwe in Korea, kitfo in Ethiopia, beef laab in Thailand, steak chee kufta in Armenia, raw liver salad in Lebanon and many others. Raw meat should be best quality (locally produced, grass fed and preferably organic), very fresh and should not be in contact with plastics. Only glass or wood should be used, because plastics leach toxic chemicals into the meat that attract pathogenic microbes.[42]

Some people are concerned about eating raw eggs. There is no need to fear eating them as long as they come from healthy chickens, which range free on pasture. Salmonella-infected eggs come from infected chickens, which is common amongst birds kept in cages by the commercial industrial agriculture.[43] Healthy chickens have strong immune systems that protect them from infections. However, it is important to understand that for the great majority of people salmonella is not a dangerous infection![44] For centuries salmonella infection used to be considered benign by the medical profession, and no treatment was needed. All you get from salmonella poisoning is a few days of diarrhoea, which cleanses your digestive system and leaves you healthier than before.[44,45] As long as you eat homemade soups and stews with meat stock and kefir or yoghurt during this infection, there will be no complications. The problem is that our modern population eats a lot of processed foods. As a result, their digestive and immune systems are not healthy; they are prone to infections and get complications from them. That is where the fear of salmonella comes from. Raw eggs are some of the healthiest foods in the world! Raw egg yolk can be compared with human breast milk: it absorbs almost without needing digestion and provides perfect nutrition for us (protein, amino acids, zinc, B-vitamins, fats, cholesterol and many other essential nutrients).[46] Raw eggs provide necessary protein for the body to remove toxic metals (mercury, lead, aluminium and other toxic metals) and other toxins.[47] Cooked eggs may lose that ability. Eating raw eggs has been a healthy practice for people for millennia all over the world. Today many people, particularly the medical profession, are afraid of eating raw eggs and cook them for a long time, which destroys many nutrients and makes the eggs more difficult to digest and less beneficial for health.

We talked about raw milk in the previous chapters. Let us just say here that raw milk is very safe to consume. In fact milk should be consumed only raw![48] It must come from natural breeds of cow, goat or other animals (not artificial breeds, created in a laboratory). The animals must be on natural pasture (with many grasses and herbs, and no agricultural chemicals), and hygiene practices must be adhered to when milking the animal. The milk must not be pasteurised, homogenised or processed in any other way. From raw milk we can make raw yoghurt, raw kefir, raw cheese, raw cream and sour cream, and raw butter. All of these foods provide excellent nutrition for us and are much easier to digest than processed milk products.

Following this programme for coming out of a long fast will allow your body to recover quickly and restore its health and vitality with ease. You will have no digestive symptoms, which are common in people who come out of a fast on a vegan programme (flatulence, bloating, abdominal discomfort and abnormal stools). If you are prone to digestive problems, introduce salads, sunflower seeds, nuts and fruit later (after at least a week), starting with small amounts. Your first introduction of plant matter should happen on the fourth day, when you make soup. Cooked vegetables in the soup are much easier to digest than raw vegetables, and they will not cause any abdominal problems. If you would like to learn more about healing your digestive system, please read my book *Gut And Psychology Syndrome (GAPS)*.[49]

Is fasting natural for us?

Regular fasting used to be a norm for humanity for most of our existence, because of irregular availability of food.[50] There was no refrigeration or supermarkets. All food was seasonal: you had vegetables and fruit only in their growing season, meat only when you had a chance to kill an animal, and eggs only in the times when the birds were laying. Food was difficult to obtain for many people, particularly poor people and city dwellers. Practically everyone had periods of time when they had very little to eat, and the choice of foods was limited. Those periods were not welcome, but they allowed people's bodies to cleanse and rejuvenate. And when people could obtain food, this food was natural, wholesome and nourishing.

When humanity discovered fuel oil and learned how to extract and use it, industrial agriculture appeared. Powerful machinery and agricultural chemicals allowed humanity to start producing unprecedented amounts of food. Never in the history of humanity had people so much to eat! Seasonality of food has disappeared: one can buy anything at any time of the year in a supermarket. Industrially produced food is full of agricultural chemicals and has a lower nutritional value. On top of that, a lot of foods in the supermarkets are processed, which makes them unhealthy. This abundance of food has become the main cause of the health crisis in our modern world.[51] Not only are people eating low-quality food, but the natural periods of fasting have disappeared. Today we have to make a special effort to fast, which is difficult and takes determination. However, those who make this effort derive many benefits for their health and vitality.

Is it absolutely necessary for all of us to fast?

If you are healthy and are eating animal foods, cooked at home from natural ingredients (fresh meat, fresh fish, fresh eggs and raw dairy) in combination with organic plants, and if you are avoiding all processed industrial foods, then your body will be strong enough to deal with common toxicity in the environment. It isn't necessary for you to do serious fasting. Just to miss an evening meal now and then may be enough, or replace a usual meal with a vegan one once or twice a week.

However, people who are exposed to high levels of toxicity (at work, through dentistry or in other ways), and people with cancer or another chronic illness may have to consider serious fasting as a way of cleansing their bodies. If you would like to do a long fast (longer than three days), it is essential to do it under professional supervision. Just keep in mind that it is vital to have a normal body weight to fast. People who are underweight and malnourished must not fast. Instead they should consider following the *GAPS Nutritional Protocol*, described in my *GAPS* book.[49] This protocol will equip your body with quality building materials, strength and stamina to cleanse and to recover.

Mark Twain had this to say about a healthy lifestyle: 'The only way to keep your health is to eat what you don't want, drink what you don't like, and do what you'd rather not.' If you feel that way, then, perhaps, it is time for you to do a bit of fasting!

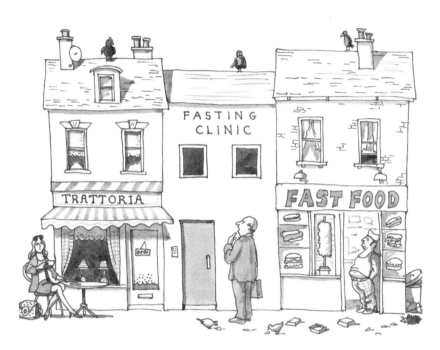

One Man's Meat is Another Man's Poison!

Sickness comes when people draw apart from Nature.

The severity of the disease is directly proportional to the degree of separation.

Masanobu Fukuoka, 1978

The human body is part of Nature! It is subject to the same laws that all life forms on Earth obey.[1] We, humans, consider ourselves to be 'cleverer' and 'more sophisticated' than animals, but our bodies don't think so. It is your own body that heals itself, not the doctor, not the medicine or anything else! In order to heal from any disease we must work *with* the body, not throw things at it or even fight it. We need to listen to our bodies. We must learn to be in touch with their needs.

Food has a profound effect on the human body.[2,3,4] Many people realise that and try to manipulate their diet in order to recover from a disease or improve their health. But, what we need to understand is that we are all different; every one of us is a unique individual. So, 'one size fits all' never works. That is why we have such a bewildering number of diets being proposed: high carbohydrate/low carbohydrate, high fat/low fat, high protein/low protein, all raw/all cooked, etc., etc.; and the interesting thing is that every diet suits some people and does not suit others. Why is that? Because it 'takes two to tango', which means that there is no such thing as a bad food per se or a good food per se, without taking into account a very important factor: *who* is eating it! Not only who is eating it, but also what state that person is in.

Let's try and understand this in more detail.

We all have a different *heredity and constitution*. If your predecessors were Vikings or Eskimos, then chances are that you will generally need to eat lots of fish, meat and fat.[5] But if your predecessors came from a Mediterranean culture or some tropical area of the world, then you will probably need more carbohydrates in your diet.[5] Ancient Chinese and Ayurvedic medicines try to classify different constitutional types, and would not dream of applying diet or herbs without this knowledge, as different constitutional types need very different approaches.[6]

Constitution is just one factor. There are many more.

Throughout our lives our bodies go through *anabolic/catabolic cycles* – in other words cycles of building itself up and cleansing itself.[7] There is a daily building/cleansing cycle, a seasonal one, and 'as-it-is-necessary' ones that can take place at any time. To build itself your body needs very different nutrients from those it uses for cleansing itself (animal foods are generally building, while plant foods are generally cleansing). Only your body knows what it needs at every moment of your life.

Depending on what your body is doing at the time, depending on the season of the year, on the weather and the level of stress you are under, your body can switch between different ways of *energy production*: using glucose for example or using fats.[7,8] Only your body knows what is appropriate at any particular moment of your existence, and it requires very different nutrients for different patterns of energy production.

We all have an *autonomic nervous system*, which is responsible for all the 'autopilot' functions of the body: for your heart beating, for your blood circulating, for your digestive system feeding you, etc.[8,9] The autonomic nervous system is made out of two branches: a sympathetic nervous system and a parasympathetic nervous system. These two systems generally work in opposition to each other providing a very complex balance in every function of the body. Again, depending on an infinite number of factors (daily cycle of activity and sleep, season, weather, stress, infection, feeding/cleansing, your occupation at the time, etc.) you will shift from being 'sympathetic dominant' to 'parasympathetic dominant'. This shift can happen several times every day, every few days or every season and it is different in different age groups.[9] The important thing is that these two branches of our nervous system require very different sets of nutrients in order to be fed: one likes meat and fat, while the other needs more plant foods.[10] Only your body knows what proportions of protein/fat/carbohydrate it needs at any given moment of your life; no laboratory or scientist will be able to calculate this for you.

Then there is the *acid/alkaline balance* in the body, which again changes all the time every day depending on many factors.[10,11] There is a myth in nutritional circles that 'being acid is bad' and that all of us have to strive to be alkaline all the time. Different foods have been classified as 'alkalising' (such as fruit and vegetables) or 'acidifying' (such as grains and meats). This is too simple. Your body shifts from alkaline to acid states all the time depending on many factors: activity of your autonomic nervous system, the type of energy production at the time, your hormonal profile at the time, respiration and kidney function, many of which in turn change according to daily cycle, season, weather and your activity.[12] Depending on all those factors, an apple, for example, which is considered to be an 'alkalising' food, can make your body acid, while a piece of meat, which is considered to be 'acidifying', can make your body alkaline. Only your body knows how to use foods at any given moment of your life; only your body has the inner intelligence to make these impossibly complex calculations.

As if that is not enough, then there is the *water and electrolyte balance* in the body, which also shifts all the time depending on many factors.[12,13] Our mainstream medicine pronounced salt to be 'evil' and recommends reducing its consumption. Processed salt should not be consumed, just as all processed foods should not be consumed. However, natural unprocessed salt (such as Himalayan crystal salt or Celtic salt) contains more than 90 minerals and not only is good for us, it is essential for our bodies to maintain the right water/electrolyte balance.[14] Then there is the myth that we need to drink lots of water every day. Different amounts in litres-per-day are prescribed in nutritional literature. Following that advice blindly can get you into a lot of trouble if your body is low on electrolytes and needs salt instead of water. No matter how clever we think we are, we cannot calculate how much salt or water we should consume at any given time: only your body knows that, and it has excellent ways of telling you what it needs – thirst for water, desire for salt or any particular food that may have the right mineral composition. Make no mistake: your body knows the nutrient composition of the foods on this planet!

These are just a few factors to demonstrate to you that no laboratory, no clever doctor or scientist and no clever book can calculate for you what you should be eating at 8am, or 1pm, or 6pm or in between. Only your body has the unsurpassed intelligence to figure out what it needs at any given moment of your life, as your nutritional needs change all the time: every minute, every hour and every day.

So, what do we do? *How do we feed ourselves properly?* The answer is: get back in touch with your body's inner intelligence! Just think: if your body needs so much protein right now + so much fat + so much carbohydrate + so much of vitamin B_{12} and so much of vitamin C, how would it let you know that it needs this particular composition of nutrients? And even if your body had a way of letting you know all this information, how would you go about providing this mix of nutrients? How are you to calculate all those factors and provide the right amounts? Well, Mother Nature is kind and it is not asking us to do anything so complicated. Instead it gave us senses of SMELL, TASTE, DESIRE for a particular food and a sense of SATISFACTION after eating it. So, when your body needs a particular mix of nutrients, it will give you a desire for a particular food, which contains just that right mix. This particular food will smell divine to you and taste wonderful, and you will feel satisfied after eating it. But in an hour or two the needs of your body will change, and that particular food will not be appealing anymore; instead you will have a desire for another food, which nutritionally will serve you correctly for that particular moment of your life.

So, the only way for us to serve our bodies properly with the right food is to be in touch with our senses!

Let us think about it a little more.

The DESIRE for a particular food

The word 'desire' has somewhat a negative feel for many people. Thanks to centuries of religious and political conditioning, desire is considered to be something we 'have to resist' and must not 'succumb' to. Yet desire for a particular food is the main way your body tells you what it needs at any particular moment nutritionally. When you get hungry, stop and think. "What would I desire to eat right now? What is the most appealing food for me right now?" Then forget about all the books you have read, forget about all the nutritional mantras about what you have to eat at a particular time of day, and just ask the question. The answer will come immediately, and just the thought of that particular food will fill your mouth with saliva. Respect your desire! Desire is your inner body intelligence talking to you, letting you know what it needs to keep you healthy, energetic and happy. If you listen to your desire every time you eat, you will be able to digest that food well and it will do you only good, because you have eaten it at the right time, just when your body asked for it.

The trouble is that in our modern commercial world people's desires for food have been manipulated through the use of addictive and taste-altering chemicals in processed foods.[15,16] Yes, many processed 'foods' contain chemicals specifically designed to make the 'food' addictive. Listening to your desire only applies to natural foods – foods that Mother Nature has designed. Stop eating processed foods and your normal sense of desire for food will return.

The sense of SMELL

Have you ever observed animals? They will never put anything in their mouths without smelling it first. Why? Because wild animals are fully in touch with their instincts – their inner body intelligence. The sense of smell gives your body a lot of information about the food. Is it safe to eat? Has it been contaminated by chemicals or microbes? Is it fresh? And, most importantly, is it appropriate for your bodily needs at the moment? So, before putting anything into your mouth, smell it: if it is the right food for you at the moment, it will smell very appealing. If it is not the right food, it will smell repulsive. Respect your sense of smell and listen to it.

The trouble is that many people in our modern world have a damaged sense of smell due to use of synthetic perfumes. All scented man-made chemicals, such as laundry detergents, domestic cleaning chemicals, so-called air fresheners and perfumes block the olfactory receptors (the smell receptors) in your nose.[17] Your nose has a limited number of olfactory receptors, and once they are blocked by a chemical, new molecules of that chemical coming in have nothing to attach to, so you cannot smell it anymore.[18] We all have met people who smell like a perfume factory, but they do not realise just how excessively they apply their perfume, because they cannot smell it anymore. The smell receptors in their nose are blocked with that chemical. The same happens with common laundry detergents, which use very powerful perfumes in order to disguise the unpleasant smell of the detergent itself. People who use these detergents regularly are unable to smell them anymore, because these people are exposed to this smell all the time from their clothes, towels and bedding. These people cannot smell their food properly either, as the smell receptors in their nose are permanently occupied by their laundry detergent. To restore your sense of smell, remove all perfumed chemicals from your environment: replace your laundry detergent with a non-scented natural one and do not use any perfumes, scented personal care products or air fresheners. In a few weeks your olfactory receptors will have cleaned themselves and your sense of smell will return.

The sense of TASTE

Food is one of the greatest pleasures of life, and so it must be! If the food is not pleasurable, then it is the wrong food for you at the moment, no matter how 'healthy' it is supposed to be! So, listen to your sense of taste and respect it. It is your friend, as it is one of the channels of communication between your body's inner intelligence and your conscious mind. How else would your body tell you that it needs a particular mix of nutrients, but by giving you great pleasure from consuming them in the form of food?

The trouble is that many people have an altered or dulled sense of taste due to regular consumption of processed foods. Many processed foods contain taste-altering chemicals, which are deliberately added to the 'food'.[19] These chemicals are not only toxic, but can alter your perception of taste for a long time, so it is essential to stop consuming processed foods in order to restore your normal sense of taste. Many nutritional deficiencies can alter the perception of taste (zinc and protein deficiencies are particularly known for this).[20] As you start consuming a natural wholesome diet, your nutritional deficiencies will diminish and your sense of taste will return. Toxins in your mouth can also alter your perception of taste.[20,22] Try to brush your teeth with cold-pressed olive oil (or any other cold-pressed oil) instead of toothpaste: this Ayurvedic procedure has a good record in detoxifying the mouth.[21] Working with a holistic dentist is very important, as many dental materials in the mouth can make it toxic and alter your sense of taste.[23]

The sense of SATISFACTION after eating

If you have eaten a meal appropriate for your body's nutritional needs at the time, you will feel fully satisfied. There will be no cravings for something else, only a nice comfortable feeling of satisfaction, which will allow you to focus on other things in your life and forget about food for a while.

It is important not to overeat, so you don't feel 'stuffed'. However, if you listen to your sense of pleasure from food, then you will not overeat, because you would stop eating as soon as the food stops being pleasurable. Pleasure on/pleasure off are the signals your body gives you to let you know about its needs. Your sense of pleasure will keep you eating as long as your body still needs the nutrients from that particular food. As soon as your body has had enough of those nutrients, the food will stop giving you pleasure. An exception to this rule is a person with cravings for sweet things.

Craving for sweet foods is a symptom of unstable blood sugar level. This problem is created by long-term consumption of processed carbohydrates, which damage our blood sugar control in the body.[20] It is essential for these people to stop consuming processed carbohydrates, but it can be very difficult for them because their cravings for sweet and starchy foods (chocolate in particular) are very strong! For these people I recommend making a mixture of raw butter (or coconut oil) and raw honey to taste. Put it in a glass jar, which you can carry with you, and eat a few spoonfuls every 20–30 minutes all day. This will keep your blood sugar level stable, and allow you to overcome cravings for chocolate and other sweet things. Depending on how damaged the blood sugar controls are in your body, you may have to eat the butter/honey mixture for a week, a month or a couple of months. The important thing is to use this time for changing your diet to remedy the problem permanently. As your blood sugar regulation normalises, you will be able to gradually reduce and stop eating the butter/honey mixture. It takes time to normalise blood sugar control in your body, and the most effective way to deal with it is to increase your fat consumption, particularly animal fats.[24] So, consume plenty of animal fats with your meals (within your pleasure zone, of course), and they will allow you to remove processed carbohydrates from your life.

So, our senses of SMELL, TASTE and DESIRE for a particular food and a sense of SATISFACTION after eating it are our friends. Let us work on developing these senses and using them fully to our advantage.

How do we apply this wisdom?

Any diet you follow is not set in stone; you have to adapt it for your unique body, for its unique daily needs. Books on diet prescribe what foods you can eat. However, when you eat these foods and *in what proportions* is up to you! Listen to your body's needs, communicated to you through the senses of desire, smell, taste and satisfaction. For example, one day you may feel like only an apple for breakfast, but next day you may enjoy a large cooked breakfast made from eggs, bacon, sausages and vegetables. For example, at one meal you were very happy to eat some roasted pork, but at another meal you do not feel like eating meat and are much happier to eat vegetables and yoghurt. Your body will let you know what proportions of protein, fat and carbohydrate to have at every meal. How? Through desire for particular food! So, when you sit down to a family meal, eat only what appeals to you at the time, and in the amounts that appeal to you.

I will give you an interesting example of how strongly our body can communicate its needs to us through desire. I know a young man who watched a film about industrial farming and decided to become a vegan. After a month of veganism, he was walking along a street and a smell of roasting chicken wafted from the open door of one of the shops. Before he knew it, he had bought a whole chicken and consumed it in one go outside the shop! This was done almost in a trance and the young man had no control over this episode. His body demanded particular nutrition at that moment, which could be found only in a whole roasted chicken. Not in a chicken breast, but in the skin, the fat, the brown meat, cartilage and all the other tissues of a whole chicken!

You are unique and nobody can prescribe the right mixture of food for you. Listen to your desire! This is your body telling you what particular nutrients it needs at this particular time. If you deny your body that need, you may get yourself into trouble: your electrolyte balance may get upset, or your hormones may not work well, or something else will not work. Remember, your body knows infinitely more about itself than we will ever know with all our intelligence and science.

Remember also that your body's nutritional needs change all the time. So, your desire for foods will also change all the time: what felt wonderfully satisfying for breakfast may not be appealing for lunch, and what was delicious in the afternoon may feel repulsive at dinner time. All these feelings are very valid and should be listened to! You are a unique individual, so what suits one person around the table may not suit you at all.

What about babies and children?

Babies and children spend the first few years of their lives learning about their environment, and food is a major part of this environment.[25] In the first few years of life, starting from the first introduction of solids, children need to develop a positive RELATIONSHIP WITH FOOD. It is extremely important to do this at this stage in their lives, because, if it is missed, then many problems can follow: not only feeding problems, but problems in behaviour, attitude, emotions and even learning![26]

When introducing first foods for your baby, remember – *all the senses of the child must be involved in the process*: the sense of touch, sight, smell, taste, etc. Our babies need to touch the food, to feel the temperature and texture of it on their fingers, the aroma and the look of it. Then they need to use the movement receptors in their muscles to transfer the food to their mouth. This must be a voluntary act, coming from the child's own decision to do that. This is very important! Then they need to smell it and taste it. Then chew and swallow. Then their body and stomach will give them feedback on how this food is affecting their insides and their whole body. This completes the experience! This is a very complex mixture of sensory input that their little brains are facing for the first time, and it is absolutely essential for the normal development of the child. New receptors, connections and centres are formed in the brain of the child during this process that affect deeply the emotional profile of this person, their general personality and attitude to life.[27]

In order to make this a healthy process *it is essential to let babies and small children eat with their hands*! In fact, using cutlery and being too intent on 'keeping things clean' at this stage is harmful for the child's development. This stage is very short, and the time of 'clean' eating with manners will come soon enough. But in the first two to three years of life being messy is the best thing for your child! By all means give them a spoon and use another spoon to feed them, but the food should be in front of the children, their hands should be in the food, and they should be deeply involved in consuming the food themselves. When the child is being fed by someone else and is not allowed to be fully involved in the process, the brain does not develop the way it should, because it receives a limited sensory input.[27] It must be a *voluntary* experience for the child, an act they are deeply involved in, for their brains to develop new receptors and wake up new centres. The same food, prepared differently, is a new experience for the child. For example, baked apple is very different from a raw apple or an apple pie; even different varieties of apples can be perceived differently. So, different recipes need to be explored and the child needs to be introduced to them gradually.

Many people don't realise just what a big part of our lives food is! And, as far as babies are concerned, it is a *huge part* of their introduction to life on this planet and their harmonious development. This developmental stage will affect the way their whole life will unfold, because it shapes their emotional profiles and their personalities.[27] If you invest into this developmental stage at a very early age, the rewards will be great for your children for the rest of their lives! Children who are allowed to develop a healthy relationship with food usually have positive and sunny personalities. Children who were not allowed to touch their food and explore it on their terms have a stifled development. They finish up with a handicapped attitude to the world and an inappropriate relationship with food, often leading to fussy eating habits, eating disorders and health problems.[27,28]

In order for the child to develop normal senses in relation to food, the child needs natural healthy foods full of flavour and taste – rich and satisfying. The food must be homemade from fresh natural ingredients! It is very upsetting to see some modern mothers working intently on their child's table manners, while feeding the child some processed concoction from a packet, instead of putting her effort into preparing a wholesome meal for her child. A mother's love for her child must flow to the child through food, first and foremost! From the moment of birth it flows through her milk. As the baby gets ready for solids, the mother's love must flow through the food, which she prepared for her child with love and care!

In conclusion to this chapter I would like to say that Mother Nature took billions of years to design the human body; it is an incredibly intelligent creation! As the natural foods on this planet have been designed during the same time, your inner body intelligence knows their composition, and knows what foods to choose for particular needs. All we have to do is treat this intelligence with respect! Use your senses of smell, taste, desire for food and satisfaction from eating it to guide you in your decisions: when to eat, what foods to eat and in what combinations. And remember: you are unique, so what suits your neighbour may not suit you at all!

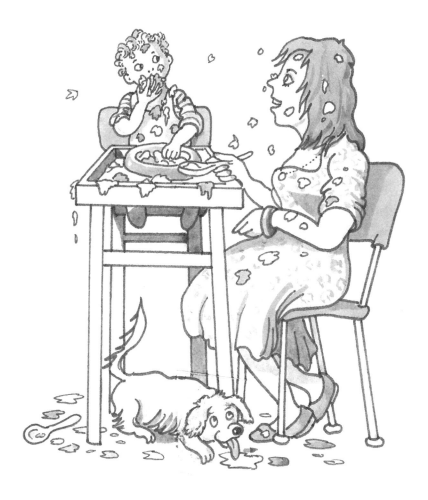

IN CONCLUSION

Nothing is more terrible than ignorance in action.

Johann Wolfgang von Goethe

There is a lot of misinformation about vegetarianism in the world. One such piece of misinformation is that you can get all your nutrition from plants. This is simply not true!

These are just a few nutritional deficiencies commonly found in vegetarians.

Vitamin B$_{12}$ deficiency is very common amongst plant-eating people, because this vitamin comes exclusively from animal foods.[1] It is one of the most essential substances for our bodies to function properly. Your brain, the rest of your nervous system, your immune system and all other organs in the body require this vitamin. Our blood composition is particularly vulnerable to deficiency in vitamin B$_{12}$, which leads to pernicious anaemia.[2] People can take supplements of this vitamin, but in order to process it properly the body requires protein.[1,2] Good quality protein comes only from animal foods, so the bodies of many vegetarians are unable to use vitamin B$_{12}$ from supplements. Our gut flora produces this vitamin, but unfortunately many people in our modern world have unhealthy gut flora, including many vegetarians.[4] It is essential for all humans to consume at least some animal foods! Vegetarians who eat eggs and dairy need to make sure they consume enough of these foods to supply them with this vital vitamin. Animal liver provides large amounts of vitamin B_{12} in combination with protein, fat-soluble vitamins and all other nutrients necessary for the body to use B_{12} appropriately.[2,3] Even Max Gerson, the creator of The Gerson Protocol for treating cancer (a vegan protocol), included raw liver in his patients' diet.[5]

Vitamin A is an essential substance for the human body. Our brain, eyes, immune system and all cells in the body require this vitamin for their structure and function.[6] Plants do not contain functional vitamin A – retinol. Instead they contain carotenoids, which in a healthy body can be converted into retinol.[7] The problem is that environmental toxins and nutritional deficiencies are able to block this conversion, so many people are unable to convert plant carotenoids into real vitamin A. Despite eating plenty of carrots, sweet potatoes, kale and other plants rich in carotenoids, these people develop vitamin A deficiency.[7] Real functional vitamin A is found only in animal foods, and the richest sources are organ meats, liver in particular. Eggs and butter also contain good amounts of vitamin A. Vegetarians have to be aware of this fact and make sure they eat plenty of eggs, ghee and butter. When you start developing vitamin A deficiency, your immune system gets compromised and you start getting infections.[6,7] This is important to watch for. The problem is that very often the immune system of vegans is not in a fit state to launch a proper reaction to a microbe. When we get a common cold, it is not the virus that gives us high temperature, headache, runny nose, sneezing and all the other symptoms. It is our own immune system that is causing all these uncomfortable symptoms because it is fighting the virus. Some vegans will tell you that they 'never get colds'. The reality is that they get the viruses, but their immune system is unable to launch any defence against these viruses. So, the person doesn't get any symptoms, while the virus just gets into the body and settles in.

Vitamin D is only present in animal foods; fish livers and oily fish are the richest sources of this vitamin.[1,7] When we sunbathe, cholesterol in our skin is converted into vitamin D. That is why this vitamin is called 'the sunshine vitamin'. Plant foods do not provide any cholesterol, so the body of a person on a plant-based diet has to work very hard to manufacture cholesterol and send it to the skin to be converted into vitamin D. Eggs from birds that are raised under sunshine on pasture contain a good amount of vitamin D. The same goes for milk and butter: the cows or goats must graze in the sunshine on pasture in order to have vitamin D in their milk. When we don't have enough vitamin D, most things in the body go wrong! This vitamin has been called a 'hormone' by researchers, because its effects in the body are so numerous and profound.[1,6.7] The body cannot build bones without this vitamin; deficiency leads to osteoporosis, rickets and osteomalacia. Every degenerative disease, including heart disease, diabetes and cancer, are linked to low levels of vitamin D in the body.[8] Lack of vitamin D is also linked to neurological and mental illness.[7,8] Vegetarians must consume good quality eggs and dairy products, and they need to make sure they sunbathe as much as possible to maintain normal levels of this vital vitamin in their bodies. Research has discovered that the majority of the Western population has low levels of vitamin D. This is not surprising, as we live in a world of sun phobia and cholesterol phobia.[9] Both cholesterol and sunshine are essential for us, but the population has been subjected to a long period of faulty propaganda against them. It is beyond the scope of this book to cover this subject fully. Please read my book *Put your heart in your mouth* to get a good understanding of this subject. Some mushrooms can produce vitamin D when exposed to ultraviolet radiation. The problem is that it is a different form of this vitamin (D2), which doesn't work in the body the same way as the natural form (D3).[10]

Vitamin K_2 comes from animal foods, and it is produced by healthy gut flora.[10] It is different from K_1, which comes from plants. K_1 is largely involved in blood clotting, while K_2 has many different functions in the body. For example, without it calcium doesn't go into your bones and teeth; instead it settles in soft tissues (artery walls, the pineal gland in the brain, stones in kidneys and liver), while you are developing osteoporosis and tooth decay.[11] Goose liver, traditional high-fat cheeses, egg yolks, butter, meats and animal livers are the richest sources of this vitamin. The only plant food that provides large amounts of vitamin K_2 is natto – a Japanese fermented soy product.[12] Vegetarians need to make sure they eat natto daily, as well as good quality eggs and cheese, to obtain enough vitamin K_2. Fermented foods contain good amounts of this vitamin because it is produced by microbes.[13] In traditional cultures healthy vegetarians always included fermented foods in their diet: sauerkraut and kimchi, kefir and cheese, fermented grains and beans, and fermented beverages.

Zinc is one of the most important minerals a human body uses.[14] It is involved in hundreds of enzymatic reactions and it is a structural element for many organs and hormones in the body. Animal foods, seafood in particular, are rich in this mineral, while plants contain very little.[10] It is impossible to provide your body with enough zinc on a purely plant-based diet! Deficiency leads to low immune status, anorexia and other mental illnesses, poor digestive function, poor perception of taste, skin problems and problems in the rest of the body. Egg yolks and milk will provide some zinc, but the richest sources are oysters, crab, shrimp and other seafood, as well as livers of animals and red meat.[15]

Deficiencies in other vitamins and minerals, protein and natural fats are common amongst vegetarians.[16] People who choose this lifestyle must study the value of foods and think carefully about what they eat on a daily basis to provide their bodies with proper nutrition. Without this planning it is very easy to develop multiple nutritional deficiencies and a degenerative illness. If you are considering becoming a vegetarian (or a vegan), I highly recommend a wonderful book by Lierre Keith, *The vegetarian myth. Food, justice and sustainability.*[17] The author survived being a vegan for almost 20 years, until she realised how misguided that was! This book will give you a good understanding of what you are getting into.

Vegetarianism and veganism are becoming popular, and mainstream propaganda paints a rosy picture of this life choice. Many people choose this lifestyle for emotional, political or other reasons, without much understanding of what they are doing.[18] Doctors see more and more people who live on plant-based diets with profound mental and physical degeneration. It is particularly sad to see young people suffering from anorexia nervosa, depression, schizophrenia and other mental illnesses because of vegetarianism and veganism. Many of these patients used to be perfectly healthy before choosing this lifestyle! Unfortunately, once they get ill, it is extremely difficult to help them.

It is very easy to destroy your health!

It is much more difficult to regain it!

Somebody asked me once: "I know people who have been vegan for a long time, how do they survive?" You can force your body to survive on anything! Let us start by looking at *inedia* – eating nothing at all. There are religious accounts of holy men and women who were reported to consume no food at all, for many years: St Catherine of Siena (died 1380) practiced extreme fasting for some 15 years, St Lidwina (died 1433), who ate nothing for 28 years, the Blessed Nicholas von Flue (died 1487), who ate nothing for 19 years, the Venerable Domenica dal Paradiso (died 1553), who ate nothing for 20 years, and others.[19] Of course, that was a long time ago and may not be true. But today there are accounts of yogis in India who apparently eat or drink nothing. In 2010 a team of medics from the Indian Defence Institute of Physiology and Allied Sciences (DIPAS) conducted research on one of these yogis.[20] His name was Prahlad Jani, he was 83 years old at the time and came from the temple town of Anbaji in Gujarat. His followers claimed that he had not eaten or drunk for 70 years. He was observed in a hospital for two weeks (with CCTV cameras and regular medical testing), and the team confirmed that indeed he did not eat or drink anything, even water, and that he did not defecate or urinate. Fasting produces certain biochemical changes in the body. Researchers did not find any in this man. If he had been eating before the investigation and only begun fasting in the hospital, then his body would have shown those biochemical changes. He insisted that he lived on prana – the universal energy field.[19,20] This study has been repeated twice. So, maybe it is possible for a human being not to eat or drink for a long time, and still live! The artist Vincent van Gogh, in the latter part of his life, was so poor that he ate virtually nothing, apart from the paint he used for his pictures.[21] It is thought that the lead in the paint poisoned him and caused his mental illness. But he was surviving! Vegans force their bodies to survive on cleansing foods only, that is why many of them look 'washed out' and are severely malnourished.

Humans can survive on anything! But I hope we are not talking about surviving. I hope we are talking about optimal physical and mental health, full vitality, boundless energy to enjoy life and be successful, finding love, building a family, having beautiful children and enough resources to bring them up. I hope we are talking about the full wonderful experience of human life!

If your idea of a happy life is to withdraw from the world and live in a cave then, perhaps, keeping your body on the meagre level of surviving is the right thing for you to do. But if you want to live in this active world and participate in human activity, you need to look after your body the way this world dictates. Your body loves you and trusts you completely; it will do whatever you demand of it. But shouldn't you love it in return? Shouldn't you treat it with respect and care? Nourishing your body properly is showing it the love and respect it deserves.

I would like to finish this book with a great quote from Weston A. Price, a wonderful scientist who at the beginning of the 20th century travelled around the world to study traditional cultures. He was specifically looking for a purely plant-based healthy culture; he did not find one! This is what he concluded: 'As yet, I have not found a single group of primitive racial stock which was building and maintaining excellent bodies by living entirely on plant foods. I have found in many parts of the world most devout representatives of modern ethical systems advocating restriction of foods to the vegetable products. In every instance, where the groups involved had been long under this teaching, I found evidence of degeneration.'[22]

Dear reader! I hope this book has brought some clarity to the subject of a plant-based lifestyle. Whatever choice you decide to make for *yourself*, keep in mind that we are *all* responsible for the health of our beautiful planet. It is our home, and we must look after it! Growing plants on an industrial scale is destroying this home. But it is in our hands to change that and reverse the process, one meal at a time.

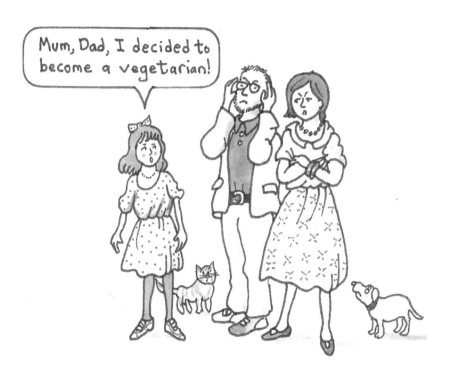

References

Introduction

1. Vegetarianism by country. https://en.wikipedia.org/wiki/Vegetarianism_by_country
2. Fallon S. Twenty-two reasons not to go vegetarian. *Wise traditions in food, farming and healing arts.* Spring 2008; vol 9; 1:37–48.

The heart of the matter

1. Levenstein H.: 'Paradox of Plenty', p.106–107. University of California Press, 2003.
2. Most packaged supermarket food is unhealthy – study. http://www.radionz.co.nz/news/national/280056/%27supermarket-food-largely-unhealthy%27.
3. Ultra processed foods prevalent and unhealthy research. http:// www.sciencemediacentre.co.nz/2015/07/30/ultra-processed-foods-prevalent-unhealthy-research/.
4. Harcombe Z. *The obesity epidemic.* 2010. Columbus Publishing.
5. Price WA. *Nutrition and physical degeneration. A comparison of primitive and modern diets and their effects.* 1938. Price.
6. Bhatia LA. *Textbook of environmental biology.* 2010. International Publishing House.
7. Sejrsen K., Torben Hvelplund, Mette Olaf Nielsen. *Ruminant Physiology: Digestion, metabolism and impact of nutrition on gene expression, immunology and stress.* 2006. Wageningen Academic Publisher.
8. Garrow JS, James WPT, Ralph A. *Human nutrition and dietetics.* 2000. 10th edition. Churchill Livingstone.
9. Hungate RE. *The rumen and its microbes.* 1966. Academic Press. New York and London.

10. Comparative digestion. Veterinary Science. http://vetsci. co.uk/2010/05/14/comparative-digestion/
11. Guyton and Hall (2011). *Textbook of Medical Physiology.* U.S.: Saunders Elsevier.
12. Saxena R, Sharma VK (2016). *'A Metagenomic Insight Into the Human Microbiome: Its Implications in Health and Disease'.* In D. Kumar, S. Antonarakis. *Medical and Health Genomics.* Elsevier Science.
13. Plant Foods for Human Nutrition. *International Journal* presenting research on nutritional quality of plant foods. ISSN: 0921-9668
14. Hoffman JR et al. Protein – which is best? *J Sports Sci Med.* 2004 Sep;3(3). Published online 2004 Sep1.
15. Enig MG. *Know Your Fats: The Complete Primer for Understanding the Nutrition of Fats, Oils, and Cholesterol.* Bethesda Press, Silver Spring, MD, 2000.
16. Pizzorno JE, Murray MT. *Textbook of natural medicine.* 4th edition, 2012.
17. Price WA, Studies of Relationships Between Nutritional Deficiencies and (a) Facial and Dental Arch Deformities and (b) Loss of Immunity to Dental Caries Among South Sea Islanders and Florida Indians. Dental Cosmos. 1935;77(11):1033–45.
18. Erasmus U. *Fats that heal, fats that kill.* 1993. Alive books.
19. Oregon State University. 'Eat Your Broccoli: Study Finds Strong Anti-Cancer Properties In Cruciferous Veggies'. *Science Daily.* 18 May 2007.
20. Ambrosone CB, Tang L. Cruciferous vegetable intake and cancer prevention: role of nutrigenetics. Cancer Prev Res (Phila Pa). 2009 Apr;2(4):298–300. 2009.
21. Cheney G. Vitamin U therapy of peptic ulcer. *Calif Med.* 1952 Oct;77(4):248–52.
22. Blomhoff R, Carlsen MH, Andersen LF, Jacobs DR. Health benefits of nuts: potential role of antioxidants. *Br J Nutr.* 2006 Nov;96 Suppl 2:S52–60. 2006. PMID:17125534.

23. Gerson C and Walker M. *The Gerson Therapy. The amazing nutritional programme for cancer and other illnesses.* 2001. Twin Streams Kensington Publishing.

24. Slavin J. Fiber and prebiotics: mechanisms and health benefits. *Nutrients.* 2013 Apr; 5(4): 1417–1435.

25. Garsed K, Scott BB. (February 2007). 'Can oats be taken in a gluten-free diet? A systematic review'. *Scand. J. Gastroenterol.* 42 (2): 171–8.

26. Cordain L. Cereal grains: humanity's double-edged sword. *World Rev Nutr Diet* 1999; 84:19–73.

27. Enig MG. *Know Your Fats: The Complete Primer for Understanding the Nutrition of Fats, Oils, and Cholesterol.* Bethesda Press, Silver Spring, MD, 2000.

28. Pizzorno JE, Murray MT. *Textbook of natural medicine.* 4th edition, 2012.

29. Ephrata Cloister in 1732 promoted celibacy and veganism. https://en.wikipedia.org/wiki/Ephrata_Cloister

30. Mascarenhas et al. 2012. National, Regional, and Global Trends in Infertility Prevalence Since 1990: A Systematic Analysis of 277 Health Surveys.

31. Chavarro JE et al. A prospective study of dairy foods intake and anovulatory infertility. *Human Reproduction,* issue 28, Feb 2007.

32. Ravnskov U. *The Cholesterol Myths. Exposing the fallacy that saturated fat and cholesterol cause heart disease.* 2000. NewTrends Publishing.

33. Caspermeyer J. *Are We What We Eat? Evidence of a Vegetarian Diet Permanently Shaping the Human Genome to Change Individual Risk of Cancer and Heart Disease. Molecular Biology and Evolution.* 2016-06-21.

34. Most packaged supermarket food is unhealthy – study. http://www.radionz.co.nz/news/national/280056/%27 supermarket-food-largely-unhealthy%27.

35. Garrow JS, James WPT, Ralph A. *Human nutrition and dietetics.* 2000. 10th edition. Churchill Livingstone.

36. Geary A. *The food and mood handbook.* 2001. Thorsons.
37. Fallon S, Enig M. *Nourishing Traditions. The cookbook that challenges politically correct nutrition and the diet dictocrats.* 1999. New Trends Publishing, Washington DC 20007.
38. Price WA. *Nutrition and physical degeneration. A comparison of primitive and modern diets and their effects.* 1938. Price.
39. Rogers S. *Tired or toxic? A blueprint for health.* 1990. Prestige Publishers.
40. Campbell-McBride N. *Gut and psychology syndrome. Natural treatment for autism, dyspraxia, dyslexia, ADD/ADHD, depression and schizophrenia.* 2010. Medinform Publishing.

Where does your food come from?

1. Levenstein H. 'Paradox of Plenty', p.106–107. University of California Press, 2003.
2. Jamison JR. Counteracting nutritional misinformation: a curricular proposal. *J Manipulative Physiol Ther.* 1990 Oct;13(8):454–62.
3. FAO (2011). World livestock 2011: Livestock in food security. UN Food and agriculture organisation (FAO), Rome.
4. Steinfeld H, Gerber P, Wassenaar T, Castel V, Rosales M and De Haan C. (2006) Livestock's Long Shadow: environmental issues and options, FAO, Rome.
5. Farm Subsidies Over Time. *The Washington Post.* 2 July 2006. Retrieved 12 April 2012.
6. Salatin J. *You Can Farm: The Entrepreneur's Guide to Start & Succeed in a Farming Enterprise.* 2006. Polyface, Inc.
7. Undersander D. "Pastures for Profit, a guide to rotational grazing" (PDF). *USDA-NRCS. University of Minnesota extension service.* Retrieved 10 December 2015.
8. Salatin J. *Pastured poultry profits.* 1996. Polyface, Inc.
9. Harvey G. *We want real food.* 2006. Constable. London.
10. http://www.foodrenegade.com/usda-guts-organic-standards/

11. Who's keeping organic food honest? http://ensia.com/voices/whos-keeping-organic-food-honest/
12. *Organic Production/Organic Food: Information Access Tools.* Compiled by Mary V. Gold. Alternative Farming Systems Information Center.
13. *10 ways vegetarianism can save the planet.* https://www.theguardian. com/lifeandstyle/2010/jul/18/vegetarianism-save-planet-environment.
14. Byrnes S. Myths & Truths *About Vegetarianism.* Originally published in the Townsend Letter for Doctors & Patients, July 2000. Revised January 2002. http://www.weston-aprice.org/health-topics/abcs-of-nutrition/myths-of-vegetarianism/
15. *Industrial Agriculture.* The outdated, unsustainable system that dominates U.S. food production. Union of concerned scientists. http://www.ucsusa.org/our-work/food-agriculture/our-failing-food-system/industrial-agriculture
16. How soil is destroyed. FAO Corporate Document Repository. http://www.fao.org/docrep/t0389e/t0389e02.htm
17. Harvey G. *The carbon fields. How our countryside can save Britain.* 2008. GrassRoots.
18. Savory A. *Holistic Management. A new framework for decision making.* 1999. Island Press.
19. Savory A et al. Moving the World Toward Sustainability. *Green Money Journal.* www.greenmoney.com.
20. Rales MJ. An inconvenient cow. The truth behind the U.N. assault on ruminant livestock. Wise Traditions in food, farming and healing arts. Spring 2008; 16–23.
21. "The Great Plains: from dust to dust". *Planning Magazine.* December 1987. Archived from the original on October 6, 2007. Retrieved December 6, 2007.
22. Brady NC, Weil RR. (1999). *The nature and properties of soils.* Upper Saddle River, N.J.: Prentice Hall, Inc.
23. De Macedo JR, Do Amaral Meneguelli, Ottoni TB, Araujo Jorge Araújo, de Sousa Lima J. (2002). "Estimation of field

capacity and moisture retention based on regression analysis involving chemical and physical properties in Alfisols and Ultisols of the state of Rio de Janeiro". *Communications in Soil Science and Plant Analysis*. 33 (13–14): 2037–2055.

24. *Water Pollution by Agricultural Chemicals*. By Dr Stephen R. Overmann, Southeast Missouri State University. http://wps. prenhall.com/wps/media/objects/1027/1052055/Regional_ Updates/ update30.htm

25. Table of Regulated Drinking Water Contaminants. US Environmental Protection Agency. https://www.epa.gov/ ground-water-and-drinking-water/table-regulated-drinking-water-contaminants

26. Change in species. The University of Reading. http://www. ecifm.rdg.ac.uk/species_decline.htm

27. Sager J. Monsanto controls both the White House and the US Congress. No matter who wins the presidential election, Monsanto benefits. *Global Research*, May 24, 2014. theprogressivecynic.com

28. Roberts P. *The end of food*. 2008. Houghton Mifflin Company.

29. India is overproducing and wasting grain now, which is damaging soil and will result in lower future food production. April 2014. Coverage of Disruptive Science and Technology. http://www.next bigfuture.com/2013/04/ india-is-overproducing-and-wasting.html

30. Harvey G. *We want real food*. 2006. Constable. London.

31. Gurian-Sherman D. April 2008. CAFOs Uncovered: The Untold Costs of Confined Animal Feeding Operations, Union of Concerned Scientists, Cambridge, MA.

32. Salatin J. *You Can Farm: The Entrepreneur's Guide to Start & Succeed in a Farming Enterprise*. 2006. Polyface, Inc.

33. Burkholder JA et al. Impact of waste from concentrated animal feeding operations on water quality. *Environ Health Perspect*. 2007 Feb; 115(2):308–312.

34. Mail Online, October 4 2016. Thought 'free range' meant

natural? How 'secret' additives are given to chickens to make their egg yolk bright yellow. http://www.dailymail.co.uk/news/article-3457452/ How-secret-additives-given-chickens-make-egg-yolk-bright-yellow.html

35. Daniel KT. *The Whole Soy Story*. 2006. New Trends Publishing.

36. Fallon S, Enig M. *Nourishing Traditions. The cookbook that challenges politically correct nutrition and the diet dictocrats.* 1999. New Trends Publishing, Washington DC 2007.

37. Fresh, Unprocessed (Raw) Whole Milk: Safety, Health and Economic Issues (An Overview) by the Weston A. Price Foundation, 2009 Posted on November 19, 2009. Last Modified on February 5, 2014. http://www.realmilk.com/safety/fresh-un processed-raw-whole-milk/

38. Dangers of Milk and Dairy Products – The Facts. By Dave Rietz. www.notmilk.com

39. A Campaign for Real Milk PowerPoint (9.4MB PPT) by the Weston A. Price Foundation, September 2011 Update.

40. Raw Milk Laws State-by-State (as of Apr. 19, 2016) http://milk.procon.org/view.resource.php?resourceID=005192

41. *Safe imports of milk and dairy products. EUR Lex. Access to European Union law.* http://eur-lex.europa.eu/legal-content/EN/TXT/?uri= URISERV%3Asa0020

42. Raw Milk: What the Scientific Literature Really Says. A Response to Bill Marler, JD. Prepared by the Weston A. Price Foundation.http://www.realmilk.com/wp-content/uploads/2012/11/ ResponsetoMarler ListofStudies.pdf

43. A campaign for real milk. Weston A. Price Foundation. http://www.food.gov.uk/sites/default/files/multimedia/pdfs/publication/raw-milk-weston-foundation-presentation.pdf

44. Schmid R. *The untold story of milk. The history, politics and science of nature's perfect food: raw milk from pastured cows.* New trends publishing. 2009.

45. Ballard O et al. *Human Milk Composition: Nutrients and*

Bioactive Factors. Pediatr Clin North Am. 2013 Feb; 60(1): 49–74.

46. Ellis, Path, Montegriffo. Veganism: Clinical findings and investigations. *Amer J Clin Nutr*, 1970, 32:249–255.

Food glorious food

1. Michalak J et al. Vegetarian diet and mental disorders: results from a representative community survey. *Int J Behav Nutr Phys Act.* 2012; 9: 67. Published online 2012 Jun 7. doi: 10.1186/ 1479-5868-9-67.
2. Craig WJ. Nutrition Concerns and Health Effects of Vegetarian Diets. *Nutr Clin Pract.* 2010;25:613–620. doi: 10.1177/ 0884533610385707.
3. Campbell-McBride N. *Gut and psychology syndrome. Natural treatment for autism, dyspraxia, dyslexia, ADD/ADHD, depression and schizophrenia.* 2010. Medinform Publishing.

Processed foods

1. Common Methods of Processing and Preserving Food. *Streetdirectory.com.* April 7, 2015.
2. Food Processing Lesson Plan. *Johns Hopkins Bloomberg School of Public Health.* April 7, 2015.
3. Levenstein H.: 'Paradox of Plenty', p.106–107. University of California Press, 2003.
4. Most packaged supermarket food is unhealthy – study. http://www.radionz.co.nz/news/national/280056/%27 supermarket-food-largely-unhealthy%27.
5. Ultra processed foods prevalent and unhealthy research. http://www.sciencemediacentre.co.nz/2015/07/30/ultra-processed-foods-prevalent-unhealthy-research/.
6. Gracy-Whitman L, Ell S. Artificial colourings and adverse reactions. *BMJ* 1995; 310:1204.
7. Rogers S. *Tired or toxic? A blueprint for health.* 1990. Prestige Publishers.

8. Rowe KS, Rose KJ. Synthetic food colouring and behaviour: A dose response effect in a double-blind, placebo-controlled, repeated-measures study. *Journal of Paediatrics* 12: 691–698, 1994.
9. Rowe KS. Synthetic food colouring and hyperactivity: a double-blind crossover study. *Aust Paediatr J*, 24: 143–47, 1988.
10. Boris M, Mandel F. Food and additives are common causes of the attention deficit hyperactive disorder in children. *Annals of Allergy* 72: 462–68, 1994.
11. Rea WJ. *Chemical Sensitivity*. Vols. 1,2,3,4. Lewis, Boca Raton, 1994–1998.
12. Guyton and Hall (2011). *Textbook of Medical Physiology*. U.S.: Saunders Elsevier.
13. Garrow JS, James WPT, Ralph A. *Human nutrition and dietetics*. 2000. 10th edition. Churchill Livingstone.
14. Mirkkunen M. (1982). Reactive hypoglycaemia tendency among habitually violent offenders. *Neuropsychopharmacol* 8:35–40.
15. Geary A. *The food and mood handbook*. 2001. Thorsons.
16. Foster-Powell K, Holt SH, Brand-Miller JC. International table of glycemic index and glycemic load values: 2002. *Am J Clin Nutr* 2002; 76:5–56.
17. Pizzorno JE, Murray MT. *Textbook of natural medicine*. 4th edition, 2012.
18. O'Hara AM, Shanahan F. The gut flora as a forgotten organ. *EMBO reports*. 2006; 7 (7): 688–693.
19. MacDougall R (13 June 2012). "NIH Human Microbiome Project defines normal bacterial makeup of the body". *NIH*. Retrieved 2012-09-20.
20. Eaton KK. Sugars in food intolerance and abnormal gut fermentation. *J Nutr Med* 1992;3:295–301.
21. Fayemiwo SA et al. Gut fermentation syndrome. *African J Cl Exp Microbiol*, Vol 15, No 1 (2014).
22. Bivin WS et al. Production of ethanol from infant food

formulas by common yeasts. *J Appl Bacteriol*, Vol 58, 4, pp 355–357, April 1985.

23. Round JL, Mazmanian SK. (2009). "The gut microbiota shapes intestinal immune responses during health and disease". *Nature Reviews: Immunology*, 9 (5): 313–323.

24. Yudkin J. *Pure, white and deadly. How sugar is killing us and what we can do to stop it.* 2012.

25. Hurst AF, Knott FA. Intestinal carbohydrate dyspepsia. *Quart J Med* 1930–31;24:171–80.

26. Fallon S, Enig M. *Nourishing Traditions. The cookbook that challenges politically correct nutrition and the diet dictocrats.* 1999. New Trends Publishing, Washington DC 20007.

27. Sandstead HH. Fibre, phytates, and mineral nutrition. *Nutr Rev* 1992; 50:30–1.

28. Freed DL. Lectins in food: their importance in health and disease. *J Nutr Med* 1991; 2: 45–64.

29. Freed DL. Do dietary lectins cause disease? *Br Med J* 1999; 318(71090):1023–4.

30. Pusztai A, Ewen SW, Grant G. et al. Antinutritive effects of wheat-germ agglutinin and other N-acetylglucosamine-specific lectins. *Br J Nutr* 1993; 70: 313–21.

31. Cordain L. Cereal grains: humanity's double-edged sword. *World Rev Nutr Diet* 1999; 84:19–73.

32. Pizzorno JE, Murray MT. *Textbook of natural medicine.* 4th edition, 2012.

33. Enig MG. *Know Your Fats: The Complete Primer for Understanding the Nutrition of Fats, oils, and Cholesterol.* Bethesda Press, Silver Spring, MD, 2000.

34. Centers for Disease Control and Prevention (1994). "Documentation for Immediately Dangerous To Life or Health Concentrations (IDLHs) – Acrylamide". http://www. cdc.gov/ niosh/idlh/79061.html

35. Xu Y et al (Apr 5, 2014). "Risk assessment, formation, and mitigation of dietary acrylamide: Current status and future prospects.". *Food and chemical toxicology: an international*

journal published for the British Industrial Biological Research Association 69C: 1–12.

36. Tareke E, Rydberg P et al. (2002). "Analysis of acrylamide, a carcinogen formed in heated foodstuffs". *J. Agric. Food. Chem.* 50 (17): 4998–5006.

37. COMA Report. Dietary sugars and human disease: conclusions and recommendations. Br Dent J. 1990; 165:46.

38. http://www.statista.com/statistics/249681/total-consumption-of-sugar-worldwide/

39. Berg JM, Tymoczko JL and Stryer L. *Biochemistry*, 2006.

40. Tran G, 2015. *Sugarcane press mud*. Feedipedia, a programme by INRA, CIRAD, AFZ and FAO. http://www.feedipedia.org/node/563 Last updated on May 27, 2015, 18:02.

41. Dowling RN. (1928). *Sugar Beet and Beet Sugar*. London: Ernest Benn Limited.

42. Altura BM, Zhang A, Altura BT. Magnesium, hypertensive vascular diseases, atherogenesis, subcellular compartmentation of Ca2+ and Mg2+ and vascular contractility. *Miner Electrolyte Metab.* 1993;19:323–336.

43. Altura BM, Altura BT. Magnesium and cardiovascular biology: an important link between cardiovascular risk factors and atherogenesis. *Cell Mol Biol Res.* 1995;41:347–359.

44. Yudkin J. *Pure, white and deadly. How sugar is killing us and what we can do to stop it.* 2012.

45. http://www.sugarstacks.com/beverages.htm

46. Tournas VH et al. Moulds and yeasts in fruit salads and fruit juices. *Food Microbiol*, vol 23;7, Oct 2006, pp.684–688.

47. Whysner J, Williams GM. (1996). "Saccharin mechanistic data and risk assessment: urine composition, enhanced cell proliferation, and tumour promotion". *Pharmacol Ther* 71 (1–2): 225–52.

48. Lim U, Subar AF, Mouw T. et al. Consumption of aspartame-containing beverages and incidence of hematopoietic and brain malignancies. *Cancer Epidemiology, Biomarkers and Prevention* 2006; 15(9):1654–1659.

49. Roberts HJ. (2004). "Aspartame disease: a possible cause for concomitant Graves' disease and pulmonary hypertension". *Texas Heart Institute Journal* 31 (1): 105; author reply 105–6. PMC 387446. PMID 15061638.

50. Humphries P, Pretorius E, Naudé H. (2008). "Direct and indirect cellular effects of aspartame on the brain". *Eur J Clin Nutrition* 62 (4): 451–462. doi:10.1038/sj.ejcn.1602866. PMID 17684524.

51. Trocho C, Pardo R, Rafecas I. et al. (1998). "Formaldehyde derived from dietary aspartame binds to tissue components in vivo". *Life Sciences* 63 (5): 337–49.

52. Staff writers (March 2010). "The lowdown on high-fructose corn syrup". *Consumer Reports*.

53. Engber D. (28 April 2009). "The decline and fall of high-fructose corn syrup". *Slate Magazine*. Slate.com.

54. Enig MG. *Know Your Fats: The Complete Primer for Understanding the Nutrition of Fats, Oils, and Cholesterol.* Bethesda Press, Silver Spring, MD, 2000.

55. BSAEM/BSNM. *Effective Nutritional Medicine: the application of nutrition to major health problems.* 1995. From the British Society for Allergy Environmental and Nutritional Medicine, PO Box 7 Knighton, LD7 1WT.

56. Gupta MK. (2007). *Practical guide for vegetable oil processing.* AOCS Press, Urbana, Illinois

57. Dam H, Sondergaard E. The encephalomalacia producing effect of arachidonic and linoleic acids. *Zeitschrift fur Ernahrungswissenschaft* 2, 217–222, 1962.

58. Pinckney ER. The potential toxicity of excessive polyunsaturates. Do not let the patient harm himself. *American Heart Journal* 85, 723–726, 1973.

59. West CE, Redgrave TG. Reservations on the use of polyunsaturated fats in human nutrition. *Search* 5, 90–96, 1974.

60. McHugh MI et al. Immunosuppression with polyunsaturated fatty acids in renal transplantation. *Transplantation* 24, 263–267, 1977.

61. Alexander JC, Valli VE, Chanin BE. Biological observations from feeding heated corn oil and heated peanut oil to rats. *Journal of Toxicology and Environmental Health* 21, 295–309, 1087.

62. Enig MG. Trans fatty acids in the food supply: a comprehensive report covering 60 years of research. Enig Associates, Inc., Silver Spring, MD, 1993.

63. Emken EA. (1984). "Nutrition and biochemistry of trans and positional fatty acid isomers in hydrogenated oils". *Annual Reviews of Nutrition* 4: 339–376.

64. Enig MG., Atal S, Keeney M, Sampugna J. (1990). "Isomeric trans fatty acids in the U.S. diet". *Journal of the American College of Nutrition* 9: 471–486.

65. Ascherio A et al (1994). "Trans fatty acids intake and risk of myocardial infarction". *Circulation* 89: 94–101.

66. Ascherio A et al (1999). "Trans fatty acids and coronary heart disease". *New England Journal of Medicine* 340 (25): 1994–1998.

67. Pizzorno JE, Murray MT. *Textbook of natural medicine.* 4th edition, 2012.

68. Daniel KT. *The Whole Soy Story.* 2006. New Trends Publishing.

69. "History of Soy Sauce, Shoyu, and Tamari – Page 1". soyinfocenter. com.

70. Endres Joseph G. (2001). *Soy Protein Products.* Champaign-Urbana, IL: AOCS Publishing. pp. 43–44.

71. http://www.alkalizeforhealth.net/Lsoy.htm Soy, aluminium and Alzheimer's disease.

72. Shcherbatykh I, Carpenter DO. The Role of Metals in the Etiology of Alzheimer's Disease. *Journal of Alzheimer's Disease.* 2007;11(2):191–205.

73. Henkel J. (May–June 2000). "Soy: Health Claims for Soy Protein, Question About Other Components". *FDA Consumer* (Food and Drug Administration) 34 (3): 18–20.

74. Messina M, McCaskill-Stevens W, Lampe JW. (September

2006). "Addressing the Soy and Breast Cancer Relationship: Review, Commentary, and Workshop Proceedings". *JNCI Journal of the National Cancer Institute* (National Cancer Institute) 98 (18): 1275–1284.

75. Doerge DR, Sheehan DM. Goitrogenic and estrogenic activity of soy isoflavones. *Environ Health Perspect.* 2002 Jun;110 Suppl 3:349–53.

76. Song TT, Hendrich S, Murphy PA. (1999). "Estrogenic activity of glycitein, a soy isoflavone". *Journal of Agricultural and Food Chemistry* 47 (4): 1607–1610.

77. Dendougui Ferial, Schwedt Georg (2004). "In vitro analysis of binding capacities of calcium to phytic acid in different food samples". *European Food Research and Technology* 219 (4).

78. Committee on Food Protection, Food and Nutrition Board, National Research Council (1973). "Phytates". *Toxicants Occurring Naturally in Foods.* National Academy of Sciences. pp. 363–371.

79. Miniello VL et al (2003). "Soy-based formulas and phyto-oestrogens: A safety profile". *Acta Paediatrica* (Wiley-Blackwell) 91 (441): 93–100.

80. Strom BL et al. (2001). "Exposure to soy-based formula in infancy and endocrinological and reproductive outcomes in young adulthood". *JAMA: the Journal of the American Medical Association* (American Medical Association) 286 (7): 807–814.

81. *Seaweeds and their uses in Japan.* Tokai Univ. Press, 165 p.

82. About salt: production. The Salt Manufacturers Association. http://web.archive.org/web/20090409144219/http://www.saltsense.co.uk/aboutsalt-prod02.htm

83. "A brief history of salt". *Time Magazine.* 15 March 1982. Retrieved 11 October 2013.

84. Fallon S, Enig M. *Nourishing Traditions. The cookbook that challenges politically correct nutrition and the diet dictocrats.* 1999. New Trends Publishing, Washington DC 2007.

85. Lopez BA. "Hallstatt's White Gold: Salt". *Virtual Vienna Net*. Retrieved 3 March 2013.
86. "Most Americans should consume less sodium". *Salt*. Centers for Disease Control and Prevention. Retrieved 17 October 2013.
87. "References on food salt & health issues". Salt Institute. 2009. Retrieved 5 December 2010.
88. Strazzullo et al (2009). "Salt intake, stroke, and cardiovascular disease: meta-analysis of prospective studies". *British Medical Journal* 339 (b4567).
89. He FJ, Li J, Macgregor GA. (3 April 2013). "Effect of longer term modest salt reduction on blood pressure: Cochrane systematic review and meta-analysis of randomised trials.". *BMJ* (Clinical research ed.) 346: f1325.
90. Graudal NA, Hubeck-Graudal T, Jurgens G. (9 November 2011). "Effects of low sodium diet versus high sodium diet on blood pressure, renin, aldosterone, catecholamines, cholesterol, and triglyceride.". *The Cochrane database of systematic reviews* (11): CD004022.
91. Stolarz-Skrzypek K, Staessen JA. (March 2015). "Reducing salt intake for prevention of cardiovascular disease—times are changing." *Advances in chronic kidney disease* 22 (2): 108–15.
92. Guyton and Hall (2011). *Textbook of Medical Physiology*. U.S.: Saunders Elsevier.
93. Pizzorno JE, Murray MT. *Textbook of natural medicine*. 4th edition, 2012.

What should we eat to be healthy and full of energy?

1. http://www.curezone.org/foods/microwave_oven_risk.asp Microwave oven. The hidden hazards.
2. http://www.naturalnews.com/030651_microwave_ cooking_ cancer.html Why and how microwave cooking causes cancer.

3. Garrow JS, James WPT, Ralph A. *Human nutrition and dietetics*. 2000. 10th edition. Churchill Livingstone.
4. Kleinbongard P et al (2006). "Plasma nitrite concentrations reflect the degree of endothelial dysfunction in humans". *Free Radical Biology and Medicine* 40 (2): 295–302.
5. "Additives Used in Meat". *Meat Science*. Illinois State University. Retrieved 16 December 2010.
6. Nutrient composition of chicken meat. 2009 Rural Industries Research and Development Corporation. ISBN 1 74151 799 0, ISSN 1440-6845.
7. Ensimger AH et al. *The Concise Encyclopedia of Food and Nutrition*. CRC Press, 1995.
8. Pizzorno JE, Murray MT. *Textbook of natural medicine*. 4th edition, 2012.
9. Stipanuk MH. (2006). *Biochemical, Physiological and Molecular Aspects of Human Nutrition* (2nd ed.). Philadelphia: Saunders.
10. Masterjohn C. On the trail of the elusive x factor: a sixty-two-year-old mystery finally solved. *Wise Traditions*. 2007;8(1).
11. Price WA. *Nutrition and physical degeneration. A comparison of primitive and modern diets and their effects*. 1938. Price.
12. Fallon S, Enig M. *Nourishing Traditions. The cookbook that challenges politically correct nutrition and the diet dictocrats*. 1999. New Trends Publishing, Washington DC 20007.
13. Cordain J, Eaton SB, Miller JB, Mann N, Hill K. The paradoxical nature of hunter-gatherer diets: meat-based, yet non-atherogenic. *Eur J Clin Nutr* 2002; 56(Suppl.1): S42–52.
14. Daniel K., "Why Broth is Beautiful: Essential Roles for Proline, Glycine and Gelatin," Weston A. Price Foundation. http://www. westonaprice.org/food-features/why-broth-is-beautiful (accessed 18 June 2013).
15. Gottschall E. *Breaking the vicious cycle. Intestinal health through diet*. 1996. The Kirkton Press.
16. Fish consumption advice from USA government. http://www.epa.gov/mercury/advisories.htm

17. Bjornberg KA, Vahter M, Grawé KP, Berglund M. (2005). "Methyl Mercury Exposure in Swedish Women with High Fish Consumption". *Science of the Total Environment* 341 (1–3): 45–52.
18. Rowland IR, Grasso P, Davies MJ. The methylation of mercuric chloride by human intestinal bacteria. *Experientia.* 1975 Sep 15;31(9):1064–5.
19. Prakash, Satya et al (2011). "Gut microbiota: next frontier in understanding human health and development of biotherapeutics". *Biologics: Targets and Therapy* 5: 71–86.
20. FDA/EPA (2004). "What You Need to Know About Mercury in Fish and Shellfish". Retrieved October 25, 2006.
21. Mercury Levels in Commercial Fish and Shellfish (1990–2010). United States Food and Drug Administration. Retrieved July 1, 2011.
22. Serhan CN, Chiang N, Van Dyke TE. Resolving inflammation: dual anti-inflammatory and pro-resolution lipid mediators. *Nat Rev Immunol.* 2008 May;8(5):349–61.
23. Pedersen MH, Molgaard C, Hellgren LI, Lauritzen L. Effects of fish oil supplementation on markers of the metabolic syndrome. *J Pediatr.* 2010 Sep;157(3):395–400.
24. Garrow JS, James WPT, Ralph A. *Human nutrition and dietetics.* 2000. 10th edition. Churchill Livingstone. Alberts et al. *Molecular Biology of the Cell:* 4th edition, NY: Garland Science, 2002.
25. Pizzorno JE, Murray MT. Textbook of natural medicine. 4th edition, 2012.
26. Porter R. *The Greatest Benefit to Mankind: A Medical History of Humanity.* 1999.
27. Gray N. "No link between eggs and heart disease or stroke, says BMJ meta-analysis." January 25, 2013. foodnavigator. com/Science/No-link-between-eggs-and-heart-disease-or-stroke-says-BMJ-meta-analysis
28. Ensimger AH et al. *The Concise Encyclopedia of Food and Nutrition.* CRC Press, 1995.

29. Sies H. Antioxidants in disease mechanisms and therapy. *Adv Pharmacol* Vol 38, San Diego: Academic Press, 1997.
30. Irons R. Pasteurization Does Harm Real Milk. realmilk.com/ health/pasteurization-does-harm-real-milk/
31. Palupi E, Jayanegara A, Ploeger A, Kahl J. (November 2012). "Comparison of nutritional quality between conventional and organic dairy products: a meta-analysis". *J. Sci. Food Agric.* 92 (14): 2774–81.
32. Enig MG. *Know Your Fats: The Complete Primer for Understanding the Nutrition of Fats, Oils, and Cholesterol.* Bethesda Press, Silver Spring, MD, 2000.
33. Oster K, Oster J, Ross D. "Immune Response to Bovine Xanthine Oxidase in Atherosclerotic Patients." *American Laboratory*, August, 1974, 4147.
34. Perkin MR. Unpasteurized milk: health or hazard? *Clinical and Experimental Allergy* 2007 May; 35(5) 627–630.
35. Waser M, Michels KB, Bieli C et al. Inverse association of farm milk consumption with asthma and allergy in rural and suburban populations across Europe. *Clinical Exp Allergy* 2007; 37:661–70.
36. realmilk.com/real-milk-finder/
37. nhs.uk/conditions/Lactose-intolerance/Pages/Introduction.aspx
38. O'Hara AM, Shanahan F. (2006). "The gut flora as a forgotten organ. EMBO reports", 7 (7): 688–693.
39. Gottschall E. *Breaking the vicious cycle. Intestinal health through diet.* 1996. The Kirkton Press.
40. Kris-Etherton PM et al (1999). "Nuts and their bioactive constituents: effects on serum lipids and other factors that affect disease risk". *Am J Clin Nutr* 70 (3 Suppl): 504S–511S.
41. Sabaté J et al (1993). "Effects of walnuts on serum lipid levels and blood pressure in normal men". *Engl J Med* 328 (9): 603–607.
42. Kelly JH, Sabaté J. (2006). "Nuts and coronary heart disease: an epidemiological perspective". *Br J Nutr* 96: S61–S67.

43. Dreher ML, Maher CV, Kearney P. The traditional and emerging role of nuts in healthful diets. *Nutr Rev* 1996; 54:241–5.
44. Campbell-Mcbride N. *Gut and psychology syndrome. Natural treatment for autism, dyspraxia, dyslexia, ADD/ADHD, depression and schizophrenia.* 2010. Medinform Publishing.
45. Fallon S, Enig M. *Nourishing Traditions. The cookbook that challenges politically correct nutrition and the diet dictocrats.* 1999. New Trends Publishing, Washington DC, 20007.
46. Els JM, Van Damme et al. (1998). *Handbook of Plant Lectins: Properties and Biomedical Applications.* John Wiley & Sons.
47. Enig MG. *Know Your Fats: The Complete Primer for Understanding the Nutrition of Fats, Oils, and Cholesterol.* Bethesda Press, Silver Spring, MD, 2000.
48. BSAEM/BSNM. Effective Nutritional Medicine: the application of nutrition to major health problems. 1995. From the British Society for Allergy Environmental and Nutritional Medicine, PO Box 7 Knighton, LD7 1WT.
49. Pizzorno JE, Murray MT. *Textbook of natural medicine.* 4th edition, 2012.
50. Horrobin D. *The madness of Adam and Eve.* Bantam Press. ISBN 0 593 04649 8, 2001.
51. Nelson GJ et al (1997). "The effect of dietary arachidonic acid on plasma lipoprotein distributions, apoproteins, blood lipid levels, and tissue fatty acid composition in humans". *Lipids* 32 (4): 427–33.
52. Kelley DS et al (1998). "Arachidonic acid supplementation enhances synthesis of eicosanoids without suppressing immune functions in young healthy men". *Lipids* 33 (2): 125–30.
53. Gupta MK. (2007). *Practical guide for vegetable oil processing.* AOCS Press, Urbana, Illinois
54. Dam H, Sondergaard E. The encephalomalacia producing effect of arachidonic and linoleic acids. *Zeitschrift fur Ernahrungswissenschaft* 2, 217–222, 1962.

55. Pinckney ER. The potential toxicity of excessive polyunsaturates. Do not let the patient harm himself. *American Heart Journal* 85, 723726, 1973.
56. West CE, Redgrave TG. Reservations on the use of polyunsaturated fats in human nutrition. *Search* 5, 90–96, 1974.
57. McHugh MI et al. Immunosuppression with polyunsaturated fatty acids in renal transplantation. *Transplantation* 24, 263–267, 1977.
58. Alexander JC, Valli VE, Chanin BE. Biological observations from feeding heated corn oil and heated peanut oil to rats. *Journal of Toxicology and Environmental Health* 21, 295–309, 1087.
59. Ravnskov U. *The Cholesterol Myths. Exposing the fallacy that saturated fat and cholesterol cause heart disease.* 2000. NewTrends Publishing.
60. Garrow JS, James WPT, Ralph A. *Human nutrition and dietetics.* 2000. 10th edition. Churchill Livingstone.
61. Campbell-McBride N. *Put your heart in your mouth. What really is heart disease and what can we do to prevent and even reverse it.* 2007. Medinform Publishing.
62. Mann GV. Coronary heart disease: "Doing the wrong things." *Nutrition Today* July/August, p.12–14, 1985.
63. Alberts et al. *Molecular Biology of the Cell*: 4th edition, NY: Garland Science, 2002.
64. Nelson DL and Cox MM. *Lehninger Principles of Biochemistry*, 4th edition, 2004.
65. Seeley RR, Stephens TD, Tate P. *Anatomy and physiology*, 2nd edition. Mosby Year Book, 1992.
66. Enig M. *Know Your Fats: The Complete Primer for Understanding the Nutrition of Fats, Oils and Cholesterol.* Silver Spring: Bethseda Press, 2000.
67. Strauss E. Developmental Biology: one-eyed animals implicate cholesterol in development. *Science* 280;1528–1529; 1998.
68. Dietschy JM, Turley SD. Cholesterol metabolism in the brain. *Curr Opin Lipidol.* 2001, 12: 105–112.

69. Moore KL, Persaud TV. (2011). *The developing human—clinical oriented embryology.* 9th edition. USA: Saunders, an imprint of Elsevier Inc.
70. Purves W, Sadava D, Orians G and Heller C. 2004. *Life: The Science of Biology,* 7th edition. Sunderland, MA: Sinauer.
71. Berg JM, Tymoczko JL and Stryer L. *Biochemistry,* 2006.
72. Huttenlocher PR, Dabholkar AS. (1997). "Regional differences in synaptogenesis in human cerebral cortex". *The Journal of Comparative Neurology* 387 (2).
73. Graveline D. *Lipitor – thief of memory, statin drugs and the misguided war on cholesterol.* 2006. Infinity Publishing, Haverford, Pennsylvania.
74. Ravnskov U. *The Cholesterol Myths. Exposing the fallacy that saturated fat and cholesterol cause heart disease.* 2000. NewTrends Publishing.
75. Enig M. *Know Your Fats: The Complete Primer for Understanding the Nutrition of Fats, Oils and Cholesterol.* Silver Spring: Bethseda Press, 2000.
76. UCSF Medical Centre data: /ucsfhealth.org/education/cholesterol_content_of_foods
77. USDA food composition nutrient database online.
78. Graveline D. *The statin damage crisis.* 2014. Infinity Publishing.
79. Horrobin DF. Lowering cholesterol concentrations and mortality. *British Medical Journal* 301, 554, 1990.
80. Albert DJ et al. Aggression in humans: what is its biological foundation? *Neurosci Biobehav Rev.* 1993;17:405–425.
81. Golomb BA. Cholesterol and violence: is there a connection? *Annals of Internal Medicine* 128, 478–487, 1998.
82. Bahrke MS et al. Psychological and behavioural effects of endogenous testosterone levels and anabolic-androgenic steroids among males. Review. *Sports Med.* 1990; 10:303–337.
83. Bhasin S et al. Sexual dysfunction in men and women with endocrine disorders. *Lancet.* 2007 Feb 17;369(9561): 597–611. Review.

84. Jacobs D et al. Report of the conference on low blood cholesterol: Mortality associations. *Circulation* 86, 1046–1060, 1992.

85. Rosch PJ. Views on Cholesterol. *Health and Stress. The Newsletter of The American Institute of Stress*, volumes 1995: 1, 1998: 1, 1999: 8, 2001: 2,4,7.

86. Harris HW et al. The lipemia of sepsis: triglyceride-rich lipoproteins as agents of innate immunity. *Journal of Endotoxin Research* 6, 421–430, 2001.

87. Iribarren C et al. Serum total cholesterol and risk of hospitalisation and death from respiratory disease. Int J Epidemiol 26, 1191–1202, 1997.

88. Iribarren C et al. Cohort study of serum total cholesterol and in-hospital incidence of infectious diseases. Epidemiology and Infection 121, 335-347, 1998.

89. Bhakdi S et al. Binding and partial inactivation of Staphylococcus aureus A-toxin by human plasma low density lipoprotein. *Journal of Biological Chemistry* 258, 5899–5904, 1983.

90. Claxton AJ et al. Association between serum total cholesterol and HIV infection in a high-risk cohort of young men. *Journal of acquired immune deficiency syndromes and human retrovirology* 17, 51–57, 1998.

91. Muldoon MF et al. Immune system differences in men with hypo- or hypercholesterolemia. *Clinical Immunology and Immunopathology* 84, 145–149, 1997.

92. Neaton JD, Wentworth DN. Low serum cholesterol and risk of death from AIDS. *AIDS* 11, 929–930, 1997.

93. Ravnskov U. High cholesterol may protect against infections and atherosclerosis. Q J Med 2003;96:927–34.

94. Porter R (2006). *The Cambridge History of Medicine.* Cambridge University Press.

95. Campbell-McBride N. *Put your heart in your mouth. What really is heart disease and what we can do prevent and even reverse it.* 2007. Medinform publishing.

96. Els JM Van Damme et al. (March 30, 1998). *Handbook of Plant Lectins: Properties and Biomedical Applications.* John Wiley & Sons.

97. Shechter Y. Bound lectins that mimic insulin produce persistent insulin-like activities. *Endocrinology* 1983:113: 1921–6.

98. Sandstead HH. Fibre, phytates, and mineral nutrition. *Nutr Rev* 1992; 50:30–1.

99. Elli L et al. (2015). "Diagnosis of gluten related disorders: celiac disease, wheat allergy and non-celiac gluten sensitivity". *World J Gastroenterol*, 21 (23): 7110–9.

100. Smith MW, Phillips AD. Abnormal expression of dipeptidyl peptidase IV activity in enterocyte brush-border membranes of children suffering from celiac disease. *Exp Physiol* 1990 Jul; 75(4);613–6.

101. Map of Life – "Gut fermentation in herbivorous animals". University of Cambridge. October 27, 2015. http://www.mapoflife.org/topics/topic_206_Gut-fermentation-in-herbivorous-animals/

102. Steinkraus KH, Ed. (1995). *Handbook of Indigenous Fermented Foods.* New York, Marcel Dekker, Inc.

103. Ulijaszek S, Strickland SS. *Nutritional Anthropology: Prospects and Perspectives.* London: Smith-Gordon, 1993.

104. Fallon S, Enig M. *Nourishing Traditions. The cookbook that challenges politically correct nutrition and the diet dictocrats.* 1999. New Trends Publishing, Washington DC, 20007.

105. Campbell-McBride N. *Gut and psychology syndrome. Natural treatment for autism, dyspraxia, dyslexia, ADD/ADHD, depression and schizophrenia.* 2010. Medinform Publishing.

106. Cooper RA, Molan PC and Harding KG. The sensitivity to honey of Gram-positive cocci of clinical significance isolated from wounds. *Journal of Applied Microbiology*, 93, 857–863, (2002).

107. Honey: health benefits and uses in medicine. http://www.medicalnewstoday.com/articles/264667.php

108. Honey kills antibiotic-resistant bugs. Published online 19 November 2002 | *Nature*. doi:10.1038/news021118-1.
109. Herman AC et al. Effect of honey on nocturnal cough and sleep quality: a double-blind, randomized, placebo-controlled study. *Paediatrics* Volume 130, Number 3, September 2012.
110. Honey holds some promise for treating burns. Published: 9 October 2008, http://www.hbns.org
111. Haffejee IE, Moosa A. Honey in the treatment of infantile gastroenteritis. *Br Med J (Clin Res Ed)* 1985;290:1866.
112. Oesophagus: heartburn and honey. Clinical review. *BMJ* 2001;323:736.
113. Oduwole O, Meremikwu MM, Oyo-Ita A, Udoh EE. (2014). "Honey for acute cough in children". *Cochrane Database Syst Rev* (Systematic review) 3 (12): CD007094.
114. Majtan J. (2014). "Honey: an immunomodulator in wound healing". *Wound Repair Regen.* 22 (2 Mar–Apr): 187–192.
115. Al-Sahib W, Marshall RJ. "The fruit of the date palm: its possible use as the best food for the future?" *J Food Science Nutr* 2003; 54: 247–59.
116. Carughi A. "Health Benefits of Sun-Dried Raisins". http://www.raisins.net/Raisins_and_Health_200810.pdf
117. Grivetti LE and Applegate EA. "From Olympia to Atlanta: agricultural-historic perspective on diet and athletic training". *J Clinical Nutr* 1997; 127:S860–868.
118. Hooshmand S and Arjmandi BH. "Viewpoint: dried plum, an emerging functional food that may effectively improve bone health". *Ageing Res Reviews* 2009; 8: 122–7.
119. Slavin JL. (July–August 2006). "Figs: past, present and future". *Nutrition Today* 41 (4): 180–184.
120. Steinkraus KH. Ed. (1995). *Handbook of Indigenous Fermented Foods*. New York, Marcel Dekker, Inc.
121. Murray MT. *The complete book of juicing.* 2014. Random House.
122. Gerson C with Bishop B. *Healing the Gerson way. Defeating cancer and other chronic diseases.* 2007. Totality Books.

123. BSAEM/BSNM. *Effective Nutritional Medicine: the application of nutrition to major health problems*. 1995. From the British Society for Allergy Environmental and Nutritional Medicine, PO Box 7 Knighton, LD7 1WT.

124. Pizzorno JE, Murray MT. *Textbook of natural medicine*. 4th edition, 2012.

125. "The Real Reasons Juice Cleanses Can Get Your Health Back on Track". awaken.com. Retrieved 7 May 2015.

126. Benachour N, Aris A. 2009. Toxic effects of low doses of bisphenol-A on human placental cells. *Toxicology and Applied Pharmacology* 241:322–8.

127. Brede C, Fjeldal P, Skjevrak I et al. 2003. Increased migration levels of bisphenol A from polycarbonate baby bottles after dishwashing, boiling and brushing. *Food Additives & Contaminants*: Part A 20(7):684–9.

128. Braun JM, Kalkbrenner AE, Calafat AM et al. 2011. Impact of early-life bisphenol A exposure on behaviour and executive function in children. *Pediatrics* 128(5):873–882 http://pediatrics.aappublications.org [Accessed September 2014].

129. CPSC. 2011. FAQs: *Bans on phthalates in toys*. Consumer Product Safety Commission (US). www.cpsc.gov [Accessed September 2014].

130. Diamanti-Kandarakis E, Bourguignon JP, Guidice LC et al. 2009. Endocrine-disrupting chemicals: an Endocrine Society scientific statement. *Endocrine Reviews* 30(4): 293–342. www.endo-society.org [Accessed September 2014].

131. Juliano LM, Griffiths RR (2004). "A critical review of caffeine withdrawal: empirical validation of symptoms and signs, incidence, severity, and associated features". *Psychopharmacology* 176 (1): 1–29.

132. Mihaljev Z et al. Levels of some microelements and essential heavy metals in herbal teas in Serbia. *Acta Pol Pharm.* 2014 May–Jun;71(3):385–91.

133. Heavy metal contents in tea and herb leaves. *Pakistan J Biol Sciences*. 2003, Vol 6;3,2088–212.

134. Vartanian LR, Schwartz MB, Brownell KD. Effects of soft drink consumption on nutrition and health: a systematic review and meta-analysis. *Am J Public Health.* 2007; 97:667–75.

135. Malik VS et al. Sugar-sweetened beverages and risk of metabolic syndrome and type 2 diabetes: a meta-analysis. *Diabetes Care.* 2010;33:2477–83.

136. De Koning L et al. Sweetened beverage consumption, incident coronary heart disease, and biomarkers of risk in men. *Circulation.* 2012;125:1735–41, S1.

137. Couzin J. (2007). "Souring on Fake Sugar". *Science* 317 (5834): 29c.

138. Puddey IB et al. Alcohol and endothelial function: a brief review. *Clin Exp Pharmacol Physiol.* 2001 Dec;28(12): 1020–4.

139. Bamforth CW. (17–20 September 2006). "Beer as liquid bread: Overlapping science.". *World Grains Summit 2006: Foods and Beverages.* San Francisco, California, USA.

140. Chopra D. *What are you hungry for?* 2014. Rider, Ebury publishing.

Fasting

1. Anthony H, Birtwistle S, Eaton K, Maberly J. *Environmental Medicine in Clinical Practice.* BSAENM Publications 1997.

2. Coleman M et al. A review of epidemiological studies of the health effects of living near or working with electricity generation and transmission equipment. *Int J Epidemiol* 1988; 17: 1–13.

3. Epstein SS. *Unreasonable risk. How to avoid cancer from cosmetics and personal care products.* 2001. Published by Environmental Toxicology, Chicago Illinois.

4. Epstein SS. *The politics of cancer, revisited.* East Ridge Press, Fremont Centre, NY, 1998.

5. Kaplan S, Morris J. *Kids at risk: chemicals in the environment*

come under scrutiny as the number of childhood learning problems soars. US News&World Report, June 19, 2000, p 51.

6. Kuhnert P et al. Comparison of mercury levels in maternal blood, foetal cord blood and placental tissues. *Am J Obstet Gynaecol* 1981; 139: 209–212.

7. Rogers S. 1990. *Tired or toxic? A blueprint for health.* Prestige Publishers.

8. Stortebecker P. Mercury poisoning from dental amalgam through a direct nose brain transport. *Lancet* 1989; 339: 1207.

9. Wayland J, Laws E. *Handbook of pesticide toxicology.* San Diego: Academic Press, 1990.

10. Fredricks R. *Fasting: an exceptional human experience.* 2012. Authorhouse.

11. Shelton HM. *Fasting can save your life.* 1978. American Natural Hygiene Society.

12. Meyerowitz S. *Juice fasting & detoxification. The fastest way to restore your health.* 2002. Sproutman Publications.

13. McKnight S, Tickle PA. *Fasting: the ancient practices.* 2009. Thomas Nelson.

14. Clinic of Dr Otto Buchinger in Germany. http://www.buchinger.de/lang-en

15. Sandra Cabot. *Juice fasting bible: discover the power of an all-juice diet to restore good health, lose weight and increase vitality.* 2007. Ulisses Press.

16. Eckhardt J. *Fasting for breakthrough and deliverance.* 2016. Charisma House Group.

17. https://en.wikipedia.org/wiki/Arnold_Ehret

18. Shackleton B. *The grape cure: a living testament.* 1972. Thorsons.

19. Gerson C and Walker M. *The Gerson Therapy.* 2001.Twin Streams, Kensington Publishing Corporation.

20. Pizzorno JE, Murray MT. *Textbook of natural medicine.* 4th edition, 2012.

21. Cummings JH, Macfarlane GT (1997). Colonic Microflora: Nutrition and Health. *Nutrition.* 1997;vol.13, No.5, 476–478.

22. Price WA. *Nutrition and physical degeneration. A comparison of primitive and modern diets and their effects.* 1938. Price.

23. Garrow JS, James WPT, Ralph A. *Human nutrition and dietetics.* 2000. 10th edition. Churchill Livingstone.

24. Masterjohn C. *Vegetarianism and nutrient deficiencies. Wise Traditions in Food, Farming and the Healing Arts.* Spring 2008;25–36.

25. Burr ML and Sweetnam PM, "Vegetarianism, dietary fiber and mortality," *American Journal of Clinical Nutrition,* 1982, 36:873.

26. Vegetarian diet in pregnancy linked to birth defect. *Brit J Urology Int,* January 2000, 85:107–113.

27. An Italian baby raised on a vegan diet is hospitalized for severe malnutrition and removed from parents. https://www.washingtonpost.com/news/morning-mix/wp/2016/07/11/italian-baby-fed-vegan-diet-hospitalized-for-malnutrition/

28. Vegan Breastfeeding Kills Baby. http://www.thehealthy-homeeconomist.com/baby-breastfed-by-vegan-mother-dies/

29. Vegan Mom Charged with Child Endangerment After Allegedly Feeding Baby Only Nuts and Berries. http://people.com/crime/ vegan-mom-charged-with-child-endangerment-after-allegedly-feeding-baby-only-nuts-and-berries/

30. Abrams HL. Vegetarianism: An anthropological/nutritional evaluation. *J Appl Nutr,* 1980, 32:2:53–87.

31. Kerr G. Babies who eat no animal protein fail to grow at normal rate. *J Amer Med Assoc,* 1974, 228:675–-6;

32. Carnell B. Could vegetarianism prevent world hunger?. Accessed on January 3, 2002.

33. Garrow JS, James WPT, Ralph A. *Human nutrition and dietetics.* 2000. 10th edition. Churchill Livingstone.

34. Cote D, Gallant M. *Raw Essence: 165 Delicious Recipes for Raw Living.* 2013.

35. Vonderplanitz A. *We want to live. The primal diet.* 2005. Expanded and revised edition. Carnelian Bay Castle Press.

36. Trivedi PC. *Medicinal plants: traditional knowledge.* 2006. International Publishing House.
37. Bushra M. *Antimicrobial activity of medicinal plants.* 2014. Lambert Academic.
38. Katz SE. *Wild fermentation: the flavour, nutrition, and craft of live-culture foods.* 2003. Chelsea Green Publishing.
39. *Physiology of the gastrointestinal tract.* Edited by Leonard R Johnson. 2013. Academic Press.
40. Fallon S, Enig MG. Guts and Grease: *The Diet of Native Americans.* 2000. http://www.westonaprice.org/health-topics/ guts-and-grease-the-diet-of-native-americans/.
41. Extreme nutrition: the diet of Eskimos. 2015. https://www.drmcdougall.com/misc/2015nl/apr/eskimos.htm
42. Anthony H, Birtwistle S, Eaton K, Maberly J. *Environmental Medicine in Clinical Practice.* BSAENM Publications 1997.
43. Egg farming: industrial versus organic. 2010. http://edition.cnn.com/2010/HEALTH/08/24/egg.safety.debate/
44. Spicer WJ. *Clinical microbiology and infectious diseases.* 2nd Edition. 2007. Churchill Livingston.
45. Ask Dr Hallberg: how dangerous is salmonella? 2010. http://www.mprnews.org/story/2010/08/24/salmonella-qa
46. Garrow JS, James WPT, Ralph A. *Human nutrition and dietetics.* 2000. 10th edition. Churchill Livingstone.
47. Naturopathic approach to prevent and treat heavy metal toxicity. Online Naturopathic Health Resource. http://www.carahealth.com/health-conditions-a-to-z/digestive-system/detox/409-naturopathic-approaches-to-prevent-treat-heavy-metal-toxicity.html
48. Schmid R. *The untold story of milk. The history, politics and science of nature's perfect food: raw milk from pastured cows.* New trends publishing. 2009.
49. Campbell-McBride N. *Gut and psychology syndrome. Natural treatment for autism, dyspraxia, dyslexia, ADD/ADHD, depression and schizophrenia.* 2010. Medinform Publishing.

50. Toussaint-Samat M. *A history of food.* 2nd edition. 2009. John Wiley & Sons.

51. Levenstein H. "Paradox of Plenty", p.106–107. University of California Press, 2003.

One man's meat is another man's poison!

1. Purves W, Sadava D, Orians G and Heller C. 2004. *Life: The Science of Biology,* 7th edition. Sunderland, MA: Sinauer.

2. BSAEM/BSNM. *Effective Nutritional Medicine: the application of nutrition to major health problems.* 1995. From the British Society for Allergy Environmental and Nutritional Medicine, PO Box 7 Knighton, LD7 1WT.

3. Ulijaszek S, Strickland SS. *Nutritional Anthropology: Prospects and Perspectives.* London: Smith-Gordon, 1993.

4. Garrow JS, James WPT, Ralph A. *Human nutrition and dietetics.* 2000. 10th edition. Churchill Livingstone. Alberts et al. Molecular Biology of the Cell: 4th edition, NY: Garland Science, 2002.

5. Price WA. *Nutrition and physical degeneration. A comparison of primitive and modern diets and their effects.* 1938. Price.

6. Deepak Chopra. *Perfect health. The complete mind body guide.*1990. Bantam books.

7. Gropper SS, Smith JL. *Advanced nutrition and human metabolism.* 6th edition. 2012.

8. Seeley RR, Stephens TD, Tate P. *Anatomy and physiology,* 2nd edition. Mosby Year Book, 1992.

9. Robertson D. *Primer on the autonomic nervous system.* 3rd edition. 2011. Academic Press.

10. Gonzalez NJ. *One man alone. An investigation of nutrition, cancer and William Donald Kelley.* 2010. New Spring Press.

11. Vasey C. *The Acid-Alkaline Diet for Optimum Health.* 1999. Healing Arts Press.

12. Pizzorno JE, Murray MT. *Textbook of natural medicine.* 4th edition, 2012.

13. Nelson DL and Cox MM. *Lehninger Principles of Biochemistry*, 4th edition, 2004.
14. "A brief history of salt". *Time Magazine*. 15 March 1982. Retrieved 11 October 2013.
15. https://www.manataka.org/page1476.html Health Alert.
16. http://articles.mercola.com/sites/articles/archive/2013/12/30/worst-food-ingredients.aspx 7 worst ingredients in food.
17. https://airfreshenerlawsuit.com/use-of-perfumes/Air fresheners class action. University of Toronto.
18. https://en.wikipedia.org/wiki/Olfactory_fatigue Olfactory fatigue.
19. Gravitz L. Food science: taste bud hackers. *Nature* 486, S14–S15, 21 June 2012. doi:10.1038/486S14a
20. Pizzorno JE, Murray MT. *Textbook of natural medicine*. 4th edition, 2012.
21. Sansouce J. Can oil pulling help you detox? http://www.drfranklipman.com/can-oil-pulling-help-you-detox/
22. Xiaojing Li. Systemic diseases caused by oral infection. *Clin Microbiol Rev*. 2000 Oct; 13(4): 547–558.
23. Huggins HA and Levy TE. *Uninformed consent. Hidden dangers in dental care*. 1999. Hampton Roads Pub Co.
24. Fallon S, Enig M. *Nourishing Traditions. The cookbook that challenges politically correct nutrition and the diet dictocrats*. 1999. New Trends Publishing, Washington DC 2007.
25. Garrow JS, James WPT, Ralph A. *Human nutrition and dietetics*. 2000. 10th edition. Churchill Livingstone. Alberts et al. *Molecular Biology of the Cell*: 4th edition, NY: Garland Science, 2002.
26. Rapley G and Murkett T. *Baby-led weaning: helping your baby to love good food*. 2008. Random House.
27. Richardson A. *They are what you feed them. How food can improve your child's behaviour, mood and learning*. 2006. Harper Thornsons.
28. Clark S. *What really works for kids*. 2002. Transworld Publishers.

In conclusion

1. Masterjohn C. *Vegetarianism and nutrient deficiencies. Wise Traditions in food, farming and the healing arts.* Spring 2008; vol 9–1;25–36.
2. Garrow JS, James WPT, Ralph A. *Human nutrition and dietetics.* 2000. 10th edition. Churchill Livingstone. Alberts et al. *Molecular Biology of the Cell*: 4th edition, NY: Garland Science, 2002.
3. Fallon S, Enig M. *Nourishing Traditions. The cookbook that challenges politically correct nutrition and the diet dictocrats.* 1999. New Trends Publishing, Washington DC 2007.
4. Albert MJ et al. Vitamin B12 synthesis by human small intestinal bacteria. *Nature.* 1980;283(5749):781–2.
5. Gerson C & Bishop B. *Healing the Gerson way. Defeating cancer and other chronic diseases.* 2007. Totality books.
6. Pizzorno JE, Murray MT. *Textbook of natural medicine.* 4th edition, 2012.
7. Garrow JS, James WPT, Ralph A. *Human nutrition and dietetics.* 2000. 10th edition. Churchill Livingstone. Alberts et al. *Molecular Biology of the Cell*: 4th edition, NY: Garland Science, 2002.
8. Soram Khalsa. *The vitamin D revolution: how the power of this amazing vitamin can change your life.* 2009. Hay House inc.
9. Ravnskov U. *The Cholesterol Myths. Exposing the fallacy that saturated fat and cholesterol cause heart disease.* 2000. NewTrends Publishing.
10. Masterjohn C. Vegetarianism and nutrient deficiencies. *Wise Traditions in food, farming and the healing arts.* Spring 2008; vol 9–1;25–36.
11. Masterjohn C. On the trail of the elusive x factor: a sixty-two-year-old mystery finally solved. *Wise Traditions.* 2007;8(1).
12. Natto. https://en.wikipedia.org/wiki/Natt%C5%8D

13. Sandor KE. *The Art of Fermentation: An In-Depth Exploration of Essential Concepts and Processes from Around the World.* 2012. Chelsea Green Publishing.

14. Garrow JS, James WPT, Ralph A. *Human nutrition and dietetics.* 2000. 10th edition. Churchill Livingstone. Alberts et al. *Molecular Biology of the Cell:* 4th edition, NY: Garland Science, 2002.

15. Pizzorno JE, Murray MT. *Textbook of natural medicine.* 4th edition, 2012.

16. Masterjohn C. Vegetarianism and nutrient deficiencies. *Wise Traditions in food, farming and the healing arts.* Spring 2008; vol 9–1;25–36.

17. Keith L. *The vegetarian myth. Food, justice and sustainability.* 2009. Flashpoint Press, California.

18. Fallon S. Twenty-two reasons not to go vegetarian. *Wise Traditions in food, farming and the healing arts.* Spring 2008; vol 9–1;37–48.

19. Sheldrake R. The science delusion. 2013. *Coronet.* pp.78–79.

20. Dasgupta M. (2010) DIPAS concludes observational study on "Mataji"', Hindu, 10 May.

21. *On the verge of insanity. Van Gogh and his illness.* 2014. Van Gogh Museum publication. Amsterdam.

22. Price WA. *Nutrition and physical degeneration. A comparison of primitive and modern diets and their effects.* 1938. Price.

Recommended reading

1. Enig MG. *Know Your Fats: The Complete Primer for Understanding the Nutrition of Fats, Oils, and Cholesterol.* Bethesda Press, Silver Spring, MD, 2000.
2. Fallon S, Enig M. *Nourishing Traditions. The cookbook that challenges politically correct nutrition and the diet dictocrats.* 1999. New Trends Publishing, Washington DC 20007.
3. Graveline D. *The statin damage crisis.* 2014. Infinity Publishing.
4. Harvey G. *The forgiveness of nature. The story of grass.* 2001. Published by Jonathan Cape.
5. Harvey G. *We want real food.* 2006. Constable. London.
6. Harvey G. *The carbon fields. How our countryside can save Britain.* 2008. GrassRoots.
7. Huggins HA and Levy TE. *Uninformed consent. Hidden dangers in dental care.* 1999. Hampton Roads Pub Co.
8. Keith L. *The vegetarian myth. Food, justice and sustainability.* 2009. Flashpoint Press, California.
9. Price WA. *Nutrition and physical degeneration. A comparison of primitive and modern diets and their effects.* 1938. Price.
10. Ravnskov U. *The Cholesterol Myths. Exposing the fallacy that saturated fat and cholesterol cause heart disease.* 2000. NewTrends Publishing.
11. Salatin J. *You Can Farm: The Entrepreneur's Guide to Start & Succeed in a Farming Enterprise.* 2006. Polyface, Inc.
12. Salatin J. *Pastured poultry profits.* 1996. Polyface, Inc.
13. Savory A. *Holistic Management. A new framework for decision making.* 1999. Island Press.
14. Schmid R. *The untold story of milk. The history, politics and science of nature's perfect food: raw milk from pastured cows.* New trends publishing. 2009.
15. Sheldrake R. *The science delusion.* 2013. Coronet. pp.78–79.

16. Campbell-McBride N. *Gut and psychology syndrome. Natural treatment for autism, dyspraxia, dyslexia, ADD/ADHD, depression and schizophrenia.* 2010. Medinform Publishing.

17. Campbell-McBride N. *Put your heart in your mouth. What really is heart disease and what can we do to prevent and even reverse it.* 2007. Medinform Publishing.